STATE $_{the}^{of}$ HEART

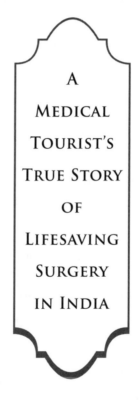

A
MEDICAL
TOURIST'S
TRUE STORY
OF
LIFESAVING
SURGERY
IN INDIA

MAGGI ANN GRACE

New Harbinger Publications, Inc.

Publisher's Note

All of the people mentioned in this book are real people. Their names have been changed except for those names made public by the media coverage of our story. The events were as I remember them.

Distributed in Canada by Raincoast Books

Copyright © 2007 by Maggi Ann Grace
New Harbinger Publications, Inc.
5674 Shattuck Avenue
Oakland, CA 94609
www.newharbinger.com

Acquired by Melissa Kirk; Cover design by Amy Shoup;
Edited by Kayla Sussell

Library of Congress Cataloging-in-Publication Data

Grace, Maggi Ann.
 State of the heart : a medical tourist's true story of lifesaving surgery in India / Maggi Ann Grace.
  p. cm.
 ISBN-13: 978-1-57224-492-4
 ISBN-10: 1-57224-492-5
 1. Staab, Howard--Health. 2. Heart--Surgery--Patients--Biography. 3. Heart--Surgery--Economic aspects--United States. 4. Medical tourism--India. I. Title.
 RD598.G69 2007
 362.197'4120092--dc22
 [B]

                    2007013005

09 08 07
10 9 8 7 6 5 4 3 2 1   First printing

This book is dedicated to my parents, Vi and Don Grace, who fostered in me the insatiable curiosity to travel to *almost* anywhere under *almost* any conditions, as well as the determination and confidence to say "I can"—and to my children, Bryan and Thane, who mastered these traits on their own, and now live by them.

This book is also dedicated to Donald Lyness (1947-2006) who, unlike Howard, did not find access to the treatment he needed in time.

CONTENTS

PREFACE: PRE-INDIA

Nothing could have prepared me for the experience that I recount in the following pages. And as with most life-altering events, I am still absorbing the lessons and insights offered to me during our pilgrimage; those that always seem to arrive as small sips over time, instead of in big gulps.

On an eighty-something-degree Sunday afternoon in September 2003, I drove across town to look at a house for sale. Earlier in the week, I had mentioned a house I saw advertised on Friends School Road to my good friend Eric. "I bike with a guy who lives on that road," Eric said. "He's a carpenter, but even if he doesn't look at the house with you, Howard might be able to tell you something about the neighborhood."

I called Howard and he offered to meet me there to take a look at the house and tell me about the neighbors. I arrived at the time I had arranged with my realtor, and Howard was just walking across the street into the driveway of the vacant house. I parked my car and got out. Howard and I stood in the driveway and grinned at each other for one of those longer-than-usual awkward moments. I imagine we were both radiant, at least to each other.

He finally said, "You should know that I stutter."

I tried to look away, down at the ground, somewhere else. But I couldn't stop smiling and didn't want to look at anything but him. "What can I do to make it easier," I asked, "look at you, don't look at you?"

He had answered this question before. "Looking at me is helpful," he said. "And try not to finish my sentences."

I nodded. "Deal."

My realtor forgot our appointment that day, so Howard and I walked up and down Friends School Road and talked for hours. He not only lived in the neighborhood, but right across the street from the house for sale, with his son, Alan. I was in between homes, happily single after one too many disconcerting endings to marriages and relationships that I'd thought would last forever. I no longer believed in forever. I wasn't looking for a partner. I was happier and more content than I had ever been in my life.

I felt so comfortable with Howard, and more importantly, so instantly attracted and deeply connected to him, I surprised myself. That evening as the sky darkened, and we didn't want to leave each other, we spoke of "going slow," of learning to be friends first, of giving ourselves time to really get to know each other. Both in our early fifties, we each had ample stockpiles of disappointments—of thinking we knew our partners so thoroughly, only to have to ask on a day years later, "Do I know you at all?" But, clearly, we were both smitten with each other.

When we finally gave in to our feelings of sudden and intense attraction, we couldn't get enough of each other. We behaved like teenagers. Having been disillusioned too many times before, I admitted to Howard that I had been sure I would never feel this way about someone again. But even in the discovery of all we had in common, I couldn't stop waiting for the other shoe to drop. It never came.

We were still giddy with adoration for each other when, after Howard went to his doctor for a routine physical, we learned about the condition of his heart. An echocardiogram showed "a flailing mitral valve with severe mitral regurgitation." Until then, Howard had been extraordinarily healthy, and he had chosen not to obtain health insurance. When we discovered that the estimate for the surgery to repair the valve would cost a minimum of $200,000, I began to look into alternatives to having the surgery done locally.

Accompanying Howard to India as his companion while he had heart surgery certainly was not in keeping with our intent of "going slow" in our relationship. But exactly one year after he gave me permission to keep looking at him while he stuttered through a sentence, we had airline tickets to New Delhi, India. My dear friend and spiritual sister, Sarina, offered to take us to the airport. "I feel like you are embarking on a pilgrimage," she said. "This journey is about so much more than Howard's heart. You know that, don't you?" Well, I did, and I didn't.

Although I understood our personal decision to seek medical care outside of the United States was our individual response to the thorny political issue of health care in the U.S., I was so busy making arrangements to leave our homes and families for however long we might need to be gone, that I felt anything but spiritual. Later, Sarina sent me an excerpt from a book she was reading called *The Life You Save May Be Your Own* (Elie 2003). She said the prologue was actually called "On Pilgrimage."

What is a pilgrimage? ... A pilgrimage is a journey undertaken in the light of a story. A great event has happened; the pilgrim hears the reports and goes in search of the evidence, aspiring to be an eyewitness. The pilgrim seeks not only to confirm the experience of others firsthand, but to be changed by the experience.

Pilgrims often make the journey in company, but each must be changed individually; they must see for themselves, each with his or her own eyes. And as they return to ordinary life the pilgrims must tell others what they saw, recasting the story in their own terms....

... It is writing that invites the reader on a pilgrimage. Because it has to do with questions of belief—questions of how to live—it makes the pattern of pilgrimage explicit. But the way of the pilgrim, so to speak, is a common way of reading and writing....

... Certain books, certain writers, reach us at the center of ourselves, and we come to them in fear and trembling, in hope and expectation—reading so as to change, and perhaps save, our lives....

... In these circumstances, their world seems another world altogether; yet they are still very much alive. They speak to us and invite us to reply, to transpose their stories from their lives to our own. That, if nothing else, is what this telling of their story hopes to accomplish—through their pilgrimage to begin to understand ours, which is already in progress. (Elie 2003, pp. x–xiv)

Only now do I recognize that this journey to India was but a short segment of our lifelong pilgrimage, which is always still in progress. It is my deepest hope that this telling finds you at the center of yourself, in the hope and expectation of examining your own beliefs, with your questions of how to live, and the choices available to you. If any part of this story leads you to a deeper understanding of your own pilgrimage and of those you love, perhaps we will all become better caretakers of ourselves, and each other, along the way.

ACKNOWLEDGMENTS

Countless people made this pilgrimage not only possible, but successful and meaningful. I especially want to thank my son Bryan Maxwell and Dr. Sakti Srivastava who were instrumental in connecting us with Dr. Naresh Trehan at Escorts Heart Institute in New Delhi. And thanks to Howard for at least *trying* to trust me so early in our relationship. To Susan for practicing her foster-parenting skills with my two cats. To my parents and my neighbors, Laura and Stephen, for keeping a close watch over my vacant house, and to Norman, for watching over Howard's.

To Jim and Wayne for overseeing the tasks at Howard's home and on the job site. To Rodrigo and Luis for keeping on; and to all of Howard's customers, especially Rachel, who had to do without Howard until he returned from India. To Sarina for the trip to the airport and, since our return, for her constant enthusiasm and steady belief in this book as a universal message for living and loving.

To Jackie, of UniqueOrn Enterprises, for her generosity in the creation and maintenance of the Web site www.howards heart.com that continues to inform and empower people around the world, and for her brilliance with my personal Web site (www.maggigrace.com) and the Web site for this book (www.stateoftheheart.name). To Kyle, Tina, and Curtis for opening their home to Alan, and to Rob, Bill, and Skip for playing surrogate dad to Alan while we were in India.

To Sally Hart for her wisdom and expertise in arranging our travel. To the ArtSchool, and to my students for coming back even after I had to cancel classes in the fall of 2004; and to the many who continue to come back.

To Bill for stepping in when Blue Cross Blue Shield of NC refused to cover the cost of my preventative "travel" inoculations and medications. To Rita, Sumitra, Deepti, and all the fourthfloor nurses at Escorts who took me in as *family* when my own was across the globe—for surrounding me with comfort and faith, and for naming things for me.

To Sanjiv, my personal lifeline, and to Naruna for managing hospitality with style and integrity. To Dr. Engel who went to great lengths to keep costs down here in the U.S. without compromising her watchful care of Howard's heart. And to her nurse, Joan, for her patience when we were uncertain and confused. To all the thousands of friends and once-strangers who clicked on the Web site, offered prayers and encouragement, sent e-mails, financial support, and a continuous stream of food (especially Jim at J&J's Deli) and chocolate for Howard!

To Dr. Mehta who allowed and arranged for the ICU nurses to bring Howard back to our own room instead of to a room on a different floor, and to Dr. K. for his personal attention. To Neil for calling on his friends in India to watch over us, and to Mahendra, Raj, and Raj's wife for showing kindness to strangers. To John Lancaster, Abhay Singh, Tim Nelson, Kady Hodges, Vicki Cheng, Suhasini, and Susan Dentzer for being careful, sensitive reporters at a time when we most needed care and sensitivity.

To all of the other patients who asked for our help and who followed us to India, for having the courage we somehow found, to get the care they needed.

To Thane, Bryan, my parents, Sarah, Judi, Donna, Joyce, and Howard, for reading the first draft of this book and offering their unique perspectives. To Jeff Olson, my agent who said *yes*, this story needed to be told, and didn't take his eyes off of it until my editor, Melissa Kirk, at New Harbinger Publications, took over. And to Kayla Sussell, editor extraordinaire who must have some functional third eye and ear to make the writing here seem so effortless. What meticulous and compassionate editors you have been.

Most of all, to Dr. Naresh Trehan, who offered us a role in the realization of his dream to provide excellent and affordable health care to patients with heart disease. Namaste. Where would we be without you? *Dhanyawaad!*

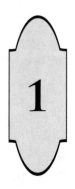

DO YOU THINK
I SHOULD'VE
PACKED A TIE?

Friday, September 24, 2004

Howard and I land in New Delhi ahead of schedule, about 10:15 P.M., to a comfortable 87 degrees Fahrenheit. We approach long lines of passengers waiting to go through customs, and then spot a sign with "Mr. Howard Staab" written in big letters. The man holding it motions for us to follow him, past hundreds of people queued up, to an official who checks our passports and visas. He tells us to get our luggage and go to Gate 5. We obey, feeling slightly guilty at what is obviously special treatment. We offer our passports to a guard at Gate 5, but he asks, "What's your name?"

"Howard Staab." It's the magic answer.

"Go on through," he says, and waves us on to a path lined with greeters, many holding up signs with passengers' names written on them. The calls and cheers are like a garbled recording. Nothing sounds familiar. I don't even feel familiar to myself. I could be watching this through a lava lamp, oily-colored and shape-shifting in "slow mo." I am beyond numb. Beyond jet-lagged. I am fascinated, afraid only of the likelihood that I will miss some pivotal handhold in my effort to understand what is going on.

When I realize the man who helped us get to this point is gone, we spot an officer with a walkie-talkie holding up a second sign with Howard's name. He follows as we walk between two walls made of people until we are greeted by two distinguished looking men in starched white shirts and ties, beaming smiles normally reserved for long lost cousins. They pronounce their names for us, but I know I will have to be reminded again and again. The sounds are not those my mouth is used to making. And I can't be sure which is the first name, and which the last—not to mention whether these men are to be called "Doctor" or "Mister" or even some other honorific title.

They take all of our bags, and we follow empty-handed to a private car that pulls up to the curb. The smiley fellow, whose name tag says "Naruna" something, answers his cell phone and hands it to Howard. "For you," he says, still smiling.

Howard takes the phone, and answers the way he would if it were my parents calling. "The flight was fine. Yes. Thank you very much. Okay, see you tomorrow. Thank you."

I still haven't formed the question of who could possibly be calling him in New Delhi when Howard looks at me and says, "That was Dr. Trehan." My surprise is not lost on him and, trying to act nonchalant, he adds, "Just welcoming us, that's all. He'll meet us in the morning." I am amazed. Where else would your surgeon call you in the airport parking lot just to say hello?

We are experiencing the kind of well-oiled plan that pulls off successful bank heists and abductions in the movies— everyone in the right place at just the right moment, handing us off like batons, without a hitch. Dr. Trehan had told me we would be met and escorted to the hospital. So far, so good.

While our bags are being loaded into the trunk, Naruna asks Howard, "Five-star hotel or hospital?"

Without looking at each other, we both answer, "Hospital. Thank you." I try to get a good look at the other man's name tag, and see that the first name is Sanjiv—at least the first one, reading from left to right.

In the overwhelming mix of cell phone calls and our intimidation, I hear Naruna answer someone with, "Oh there will be Indian press too. They are the first Americans to come."

Howard and I look at each other. The first? I think back to all the testimonials I read on the Escorts' Web site—the one woman's picture I can recall was British. It had never occurred to me to contact former patients or even to count Americans. Shoddy research! In-a-hurry research! Howard leans over to me and whispers, "Do you think I should've packed a tie?"

I pick up some mention of a forty-minute drive to wher- ever we are going; the hospital, I assume. I wonder if they will admit Howard and send me out to find a hotel. This part of the plan, actually anything beyond being met at the airport, is an unknown. We usually make more detailed arrangements when we travel, but we had other more pressing issues to focus on.

Sanjiv is our driver. Howard and I huddle in the back of a small Toyota SUV while Naruna rides shotgun. Who would have thought? Who could have predicted that I would snuggle up to this man in New Delhi, India, on a steamy night only one year after I met him? So much for our admirable intentions "to go slow" in our new relationship. We had not moved in together, and we intentionally spent time apart in what we'd decided was a mature effort to savor each moment, to continue to pay attention to each other, and to protect our unexpected love for each other from time's complacency.

I remember returning from an out-of-town week-long workshop and driving directly to Howard's house. When I walked in the door, we stood there, the way we had stood in the driveway of the vacant house the day we met, just smiling at each other. I thought he might be able to hear my heart pounding. My body felt simultaneously limp and electric. Was this even possible at my age? "I missed you so much," I said. "I could hardly make myself stay at the workshop."

He nodded. "I know. Me too."

"What are we going to do?" I asked. I felt so desperate, so absolutely sixteen and so desperately in love.

"We're going to continue loving each other." And we held onto each other longer than I can remember hugging anyone since I rocked or walked my babies to sleep.

And I hold onto Howard now, in the middle of the night in India. Sanjiv drives with his brights on. He taps the horn repeatedly, more as a general warning than at anyone in particular. It is darker in the streets than seems possible with this much traffic; certainly darker than seems safe for the bicycles and open-sided motorized rickshaws I see moving among the cars.

I try to make out which side of the street we are driving on, but it is not clear. There are no identifiable lanes; whichever way I look, traffic is moving slowly in every direction. I want to talk to Howard about the "first Americans" bit, but don't want to miss anything. I see freeway signs above, and tiny red lights along the sides. Forcing my eyes to focus, I see that these lights are fires, some with cooking pots on top, and people huddling together under tarps.

These scenes remind me of music festivals where people camp on top of each other, sharing meals they cook over Coleman stoves. On either side of our car are stray sheep, dogs loose in the street, trucks top-heavy with burlap-wrapped loads, some with young men perched on top, and then ... a cow. Many cows.

I whisper to Howard, "What if they hadn't met us and we had to find a hotel?"

"I wouldn't know where to start," and he sandwiches my hand in both of his.

Sanjiv pulls the car up to a circular entrance of what we assume is Escorts Heart Institute. Attendants who greet our car shoo us away from collecting our bags, and we follow Sanjiv into the dark lobby. It is quiet, but dozens and dozens of people lay sleeping, sprawled all over the chairs and benches and in the hallways on the floor. The first image that comes to me is the aftermath of a random shooting spree. Then I wonder if all these people are waiting for surgery the way I imagine they might wait in shelters during the day for food. Later, I learn they are family members who, in the United States, would be asleep in nearby hotels.

We follow Naruna and Sanjiv through and around the dreaming bodies. In the mottled darkness, the walls and floor seem to give off a tiny glint. There are guards or security officers at every corner, at every elevator door, on every floor. They salute as we pass.

The elevator doors open on the fourth floor to a nurses' station where a row of smiling nurses in white uniforms greet us. Maybe they have a song prepared? We nod, and keep following Naruna and Sanjiv to a private room, larger than our living room back home. There is a separate bathroom, a regular hospital bed and end tables on one wall, and a long black sofa set against a backdrop—an enormous window that looks out at our new twinkling city.

We turn around to discover that several nurses have joined us. Naruna offers us tea and coffee and points to a basket of fruit and plate of cookies on the bedside table. Somehow in these dizzying first moments, we accumulate a handful of business cards with unpronounceable names and instructions as to who will help us with what. I know I'll never remember. I clutch the cards. I still wouldn't dare say Naruna and Sanjiv's names out loud. They have prepared for our arrival. It all unfolds and feels like ceremony, as if we are important ambassadors.

One nurse takes out a folded white hospital gown and lays it on the bed. "For Mr. Howard," she says to him and steps back in line.

Another nurse moves closer to the sofa and looks at me and asks, "This is okay for you?"

"Oh, yes. Of course."

Another reality check: Howard and I will not be sleeping together in the same bed again for at least a week; we won't be able to fall asleep holding on to each other unless I climb into his bed beside him. We have arrived. The nurse takes a sheet and pillow out of the closet and places it on the end of the sofa for me. I am grateful that I will not be hunting for a hotel tonight.

Naruna asks what time we would like to get up in the morning. In some collection of suggestions, it is decided. Breakfast at eight. Naruna and Sanjiv shake our hands and wish us a good night's sleep. I am at once looking forward to being able to speak to Howard in private, and nervous about their leaving. We have been so completely taken care of. But when they leave, two nurses remain. The buddy system is alive and well in India. I hope we don't scare them, being so tall, so white. One points to the hospital gown on the bed. "Please put on. The doctor comes. Then you sleep. Yes?" The nurses leave together.

I look at Howard. "But on the phone, Dr. Trehan said he would see us in the morning, didn't he?"

Howard shrugs. While Howard changes, I use the bathroom. In a spotless tiled shower stall there are two pink buckets and a chair, no curtain—more to learn. When I come back into the room, Howard is in a white karate outfit. With his long brown hair and late summer tan, he is a striking image. He holds his hands in front of his chest like he is praying. "What do you think?"

"Is that the hospital gown?" I ask.

"Guess so." He pulls me close to him. Feeling his body through the crisp white cotton is a mixed sensation of comfort and warning. Howard is a T-shirt kind of guy.

"We made it," I say. I step back, position my hands midair, perpendicular to each other in a T, and say, "Just don't try any moves on me, mister."

A young doctor knocks and comes into the room, followed by the same two nurses who had just left. He introduces himself to Howard—yet another name lost on us. "I will examine you tonight. Tomorrow, you have more tests."

Howard lies down on his bed. I sit on the sofa, my back to the window, to a country I still haven't seen. I calculate it is two days later than when we left North Carolina. The doctor asks him questions about pain, shortness of breath, fatigue, while the nurses take his temperature, blood pressure, and pulse—all the usual. Then another knock on the door and a different nurse wheels in a portable machine of some kind. I look at the clock. It is midnight. While the doctor listens to Howard's heart, I realize we haven't been to any kind of admissions office to sign any paperwork. We haven't paid anyone a cent. In fact, no one has even asked my name, and I am to sleep in this hospital room. Why, we could be anybody!

"We do EKG," the doctor says, "then you sleep." When he attaches the little white stick-on patches to Howard's chest, my reality-check alarm goes off again. We are here to have Howard's heart repaired. Here, in India. This is for real.

When the EKG is finished, the doctor stands and removes his gloves. "All right. Only one cup of tea in the morning," he says to Howard. "Dr. Trehan has ordered more tests. Good night."

Saturday, September 25, 2004

In the glare of morning, after a few hours of deep and restful sleep, I fold up my sheet and dress quickly.

"How did you sleep?" I ask Howard.

"Quickly," he says. Howard never has any trouble falling asleep, anytime, and just about anywhere. But he wakes up early, usually before the sun, and simply knows he has finished sleeping. I am the opposite—never a napper, I am a lover of those late night hours when the phone stops ringing, and I can paint or write uninterrupted. And I adore the luxury of falling back to sleep in the morning over and over again. I know there will be none of that here, until maybe next week when we are out on our own, lying on some beach somewhere, recovering.

I turn around on the sofa that is my bed. Our window shows a wide panorama of green treetops, blooming branches, and distant buildings. I look down four floors, to the street outlined by a thick gray wall on the far side that separates us from what looks like the grounds of a school or another hospital. Bicycle-powered rickshaws (if my father were here, he would begin singing "Surrey with the Fringe on Top"— minus the fringe), regular cars, pedestrians, and little green buggy-cars I learn are called auto-rickshaws, all make their own path wherever they find room.

A young man in a vest and tie comes in with a tray of coffee and tea. He sets it on Howard's bedside tray-table, then rolls the table over near the sofa where I am perched looking out. "Mr. Howard, one cup of tea only." Smiling and with a respectful nod, he then asks what I would like for breakfast. Normally, I have coffee, and without knowing the options here, I am at a loss for words. He suggests an omelet, eggs and toast, but I shake my head. "This is fine. Thank you. Coffee is fine."

Howard has his one cup of tea, and I have coffee with hot milk. But evidently coffee is not considered breakfast here. Maybe ten minutes later, a different server in a teal jacket comes in to replace the coffee and tea with a new tray of food for me. He smiles, nods, and keeps smiling, staring a bit longer than seems necessary. I wonder how we must look to these dark-eyed smiling people with hair like liquid obsidian. He closes the door behind him.

"Only one cup of tea," I remind Howard. He is the earliest breakfast eater I know, often getting up at 4:00 or 5:00 A.M., without an alarm clock. Together we explore the foil-covered containers on my tray: orange juice, sliced papaya, a bowl of dry cornflakes, and a thermos of hot milk. "They already took the coffee away," Howard asks. "What do you think the hot milk's for?" This morning I learn to eat cold cereal with hot milk.

By 9:00, a man in a turban arrives to welcome Howard. He introduces himself as the Chief Administrator, and Howard introduces me to him. The Chief points to a tent card on the counter, like the ones left by housekeeping in motel rooms that say, "This room was cleaned by Hazel." "This is my mobile number," he says. "Please call me if you have any needs. Any needs at all." We nod, and join in the smiling until he is gone.

"I wonder if I'm moving to a hotel today," I say to Howard. "I don't want to leave."

"I think you can stay right there on the couch," Howard says. "Did you sleep okay?"

"Sure. I just don't know where they plan on my staying after today."

We both go over to kneel on the sofa with our backs to the room and watch the street below fill in with color like a fund-raising thermometer. Vendors wheel their carts and wagons piled high with fruit to park against the gray wall. Scruffy dogs wander along following scents, noses to the ground. And here come the cows in a long line. A shepherd follows them wielding a stick. Dump trucks loaded with demo'd building materials steer around the cows.

We take particular note of the bicyclist with a stack of bricks tied to the bike's back bumper, and those who ride hugging a couple of 2 x 4s close to their sides. Since Howard is a builder, we joke about going home with new instructions for Howard's construction crew. "Guys, from now on, it's two boards per trip," Howard shouts into stacked fists as if he is calling orders into a bullhorn. "Pump up those bike tires, we've got bricks to haul. But whatever you do, remember the cows have the right of way!"

Our next visitor is another bundle of smiles—Sister Rita, nursing supervisor, her name tag says. She extends her hand to each of us, welcoming us. Her eyes shine behind her black-framed eyeglasses. "Did you take breakfast?" she asks only me. I nod. "And are you comfortable, Mr. Howard?"

"Oh yes, very comfortable. Thank you," he says.

"You may eat after the tests," she says. "Please let us know if you need anything."

This stream of warm, friendly greeters continues, sprinkled with kitchen and maintenance staff. The man in the teal jacket comes in to remove my breakfast tray. A thin man dressed all in black comes in with a rainbow-colored feather duster and squats down, his feet flat on the floor. Beginning at one corner of the room, and moving under the sofa, the bed, the chair, and all the way out to the hallway, he dusts the floor in broad gathering sweeps.

Another man in pressed black dress pants enters silently. He carries a pump-spray machine and a flyswatter. As he inspects the edges of the room, the ceiling, and all around the window, we detect a faint odor of pesticide, though he never sprays. Everyone is kind and respectful. Everything is immaculate.

A different doctor who speaks fluent English comes in to talk to Howard. They exchange Southern niceties, and we learn that he trained in Alabama. He asks Howard to return to his bed so that he can examine him. I resume my perch on the black sofa to watch and take notes. He asks many of the same medical history questions and listens to Howard's heart. Then I watch the doctor's slender fingers, his skin as smooth and soft as if he wears tawny kid gloves, while he measures with his hand the distance from under Howard's left arm to where I imagine the heart's mitral valve might be.

This young doctor has three rings on his right hand, and I assume each carries meaning: on his index finger he wears a diamond; on his middle finger, a ruby; and on his pinky, he wears a pearl. He listens to Howard's heart again with his stethoscope. Then with a tender gesture, he puts each of Howard's hands in his, and turns each hand over and back again. I assume he is looking for swelling or discoloration—"clubbing," I think they call it. He explains that Howard will be repeating an echocardiogram now like the one that first named Howard's diagnosis. We come to call him the "echo expert"; then, out of sheer laziness, we don't learn how to pronounce his Indian name; we simply call him "Dr. Echo." I attribute his willingness to be kind to us to his youth and, perhaps, lower rank, but he wins my confidence immediately.

By 10:30 A.M., yet another doctor stops by to examine Howard. I keep expecting Dr. Trehan to come in, but this one is a cardiologist who wears a red string bracelet on his right wrist. Howard introduces him to me, and without explaining, I know that Howard doesn't want me to be invisible to these doctors who do not automatically include me in their greetings. He feels Howard's neck, chest, back, and hands again, then listens to Howard's heart. "We will repeat the echo first," he says, removing the stethoscope from his ears. "Then we will put a flexible tube down through your esophagus into your stomach to get a closer look at your heart's valves." Howard nods.

"Is this the TEE?" I ask, remembering that we cancelled the transesophageal echocardiogram (TEE) and catheterization scheduled back home when Dr. Engel assured us that Dr. Trehan would want to perform his own TEE before operating on Howard.

The cardiologist stops, and actually makes eye contact with me. "Yes, the TEE."

He turns back to Howard. "We will pre-medicate you for this, so you will be more comfortable."

"How long does the TEE take?" I ask, wondering if it is done in the Operating Room or in X-ray, or here in Howard's room.

"It takes only half an hour to forty-five minutes," he says, looking at Howard. "Then we will discuss strategies."

Finally, Howard and I are alone. His medical care has begun. Everything else is secondary. There is no place to hide from the decision we have made to come to India, and I am surprisingly confident. I hope Howard is, too. I walk over to his bed as he sits up on the edge. "How ya' feeling 'bout all this attention?" I ask, going for a light Southern accent.

He looks at me and his eyes soften, the way I remember they softened the first time he tried to tell me how different he felt our relationship was from his previous ones.

"Have you noticed how much these doctors touch me?" My face must register shock, because he is quick to say, "No, no! Not in a bad way. I mean, they use their hands so much more than American doctors. They touch and feel and hold, and then use instruments." He shakes his head and smiles. "It's so different, so much more hands-on."

Just then, two nurses walk in, one dressed in a white uniform, one in brown. "I put in IV," the nurse in white says, "then we go to lab. Okay?" The first name on her name tag says Reena. She is silent as she inserts an access port for the

IVs Howard will need, and when she is finished, a young man appears pushing an empty wheelchair.

The other nurse turns to me and asks, "You come?"

I jump up, fearing they will take Howard away for hours and leave me looking out this window. "Yes, yes, thank you." I learn her name is Sheela.

We make our way through the hallways we must have traveled through last night, but now it is a sunny morning. My mother was right: Everything *does* look better in the daytime. It is Saturday. We have been here less than twelve hours, and the tests we had scheduled at home for two weeks from now will all be completed today.

In the elevator, two male doctors get on—one in white, the other in a blue coat. Naturally, I wonder about the significance of uniforms. They hold hands, talking intently, and get off on the second floor, still holding hands as they walk. We go first to the Echo Lab in what must be the basement. The nurse motions for me to wait outside. Sheela wheels Howard in.

There are so many patients everywhere, I'm sure Howard is getting preferential treatment. It's awkward standing in the hallway, the only white person anywhere in view. But I try to smile and take in as much as I can, so I can describe it to Howard later. On one wall outside the Ultrasound Department, a sign in English catches my eye. It says: "Here, pre-natal sex determination (boy or girl) before birth is not done; it is a punishable act."

I think of my friends who learn the sex of their unborn child ahead of time, and choose the baby's name and the colors for the nursery long before the birth. I never wanted to ruin the surprise and magic of my two children's births, and I made my midwife promise not to tell me even if she knew from the ultrasounds. I think about it a bit more and recognize that here, this punishable act has nothing to do with interior decorating or name selection. A chill travels down through my body, remembering stories of the Chinese discarding their newborn female infants.

Sheela and Reena, the two nurses (or sisters, as they are called here), join me in the hallway, smiling a lot, but obviously feeling as awkward as I do about making small talk in a language other than their own. Finally, I ask about the red mark on their foreheads. "Does this mean you are married?" I ask, pointing to the space between my eyebrows on the bridge of my nose.

"No. No." They both giggle. "The mark here is for married woman," Sheela tells me, indicating a path up into her hairline where a center part would be. "It is dye. This one is ..." she giggles again, and gently tosses her head, "... decoration."

"Oh, like jewelry?" I ask, fingering my earrings. I play charades when I speak, even though they probably understand every word I say.

"Yes. This one you take away. Can wear different one every day."

I nod. All this time I thought the blood-red mark was like a tattoo, but it is just a peel-off sticker! I look around at the women in the hallway for other examples. Many young women don't have any mark at all, so I assume they're not married and do not choose to wear the sticker.

Suddenly, the lights go out. No one seems to notice, and they all continue on their paths in half-lit halls.

Against one alcove wall I read another sign:

▪ Quality Policy

Escorts Heart Institute and Research Center is committed to deliver the highest quality health care to Enhance Patient Satisfaction and meet their expectations through Well-Defined Quality Systems, World-Class Professionals, State of Art Technology, Humane and Compassionate Care.

I hope their surgeons are as thorough and top quality as their Quality Policy is.

In practically no time at all, Howard is wheeled out of the Ultrasound/Echo Lab. Another doctor joins us in the hallway. His name tag reads "Dr. K. ... something too long to pronounce, Head of Cardiology. Dr. K. to us, from now on.

He speaks to Howard, and again, Howard introduces him to me. Like it or not, these doctors are going to have to get used to talking to me. We might as well get started. Dr. K. turns out to be no challenge at all—he explains everything to both of us. He even adds the fact that he knows the chief of noninvasive cardiology at Duke University Medical Center, a few miles from our home.

I recall Dr. Engel, Howard's cardiologist, mentioning his name when she described the two methods of operating: by cutting the sternum or by entering through the ribs (intercostally). She had also mentioned that the expert in the intercostal technique was at Duke, but we never got far enough along to actually meet any surgeons.

Dr. K. explains that everything will be done today so they will have all the information for surgery on Monday. Again, I am amazed at the efficiency. In the U.S., Dr. Engel had to postpone Howard's TEE an extra week, after we'd already been waiting for the appointment scheduled for two weeks away.

Reena pushes Howard in his wheelchair, and Sheela and I follow to a different hallway. Sanjiv, our driver from last night, appears and asks if I need anything. When I shake my head, he asks again, "Water?" Then I realize how hot and dry I am, and look around for a drinking fountain. "Yes, please."

"We will get you water," Sanjiv says. "And what will you like for lunch?"

Again, I have no idea as to what the choices might be. "Indian or Continental?" Sanjiv asks.

"Oh, Indian, please," I say.

"Indian," Sanjiv nods. "Good. Veg or non-veg?"

I recognize this choice from my son Bryan's e-mails to me from India only a month before, and am grateful that I can answer. "Veg please. Thank you."

Just then a young man appears from the open elevator door holding up a round tray with a liter of bottled water and one small glass. He is dressed in the same teal vest as the food and beverage men. He lowers the tray to waist-height, pours a glass of water, and hands it to me. I drink it quickly and put the glass back on his tray. He pours again, and I drink. I had no idea I was so thirsty.

Here I stand in the hallway with one man taking my lunch order and another pouring glasses of water for me as quickly as I can down them. I think of Princess Di. What an odd thing to have people anticipate your needs before you even realize them yourself. But I fear I am the only one here being served in this way, and guilt creeps in again.

Sanjiv asks, "Some dal? Rice and salad? Okay?"

"Yes, that would be fine," I say.

"Your lunch will be ready when you return to your room."

All I know to say is, "Thank you very much."

Howard leaves to have his TEE, and Sheela directs me to the Pulmonary Laboratory, and then to a chair in a small office. I am to wait here. I feel like a voyeur as the lab technician reads test results from a machine's printouts—not that I understand a word. Then a patient comes in; an older woman. She breathes into a tube, following the technician's instructions in Hindi, which I imagine to be something like, "Deep breath. Now blow quickly." "Hold it," and "Now kazoo as hard as you can."

I am glad Howard has nothing wrong with his lungs and won't have to follow these directions. I try not to stare while the patient completes her test only a couple of feet away from me. I watch doctors discuss something in the hallway just outside. (I wonder if HIPAA [Health Insurance Portability and Accountability Act], our new patient portability act, ever considered this way to ensure patient privacy—all doctors must speak in Hindi.)

The patient finishes and leaves. I am increasingly anxious. Then suddenly Howard appears in the doorway. The technician I've been watching says "Come," and motions for Howard to get up and sit before her machine. She speaks in English, explains that he will now have a lung function test. She asks him to breathe slowly, regularly, then deep exhales, deep inhales, then fast breathing. Howard even kazoos into the tube! He did so much better than the older woman; I am proud of him and clap quietly. He glances sideways at me, probably wondering how I can evaluate his performance. Of course, I can't.

Then, Howard leaves for the TEE where he will be "pre-medicated," as the doctor said. This is the procedure where they shove a tube down the throat, the patient tries to gag, and if they get past that part, they will take pictures of Howard's heart to actually see the valve Dr. Trehan will operate on.

I remember Dr. Engel explaining the gagging part, and why it would be better if she sedated him. I guessed then that it would help him gag quietly so he wouldn't cause a scene. Sheela shows me to the regular waiting room, and I am happy to leave this woman's tiny office. I want to wait where the other people wait. I am fascinated, riveted by their natural, quiet beauty.

When Howard is wheeled out again, Dr. K. is behind him and says, "We did not need to sedate him. He did very well." Howard looks at me, and then breaks into a fake dramatic gag, holding his throat. Everyone looks at each other, I roll my eyes, and we all laugh. The TEE is over.

We return to our room and one lunch tray filled with plates covered in silver lids—many more dishes than dal, rice, and salad would require. Howard is still not allowed to eat because of the catheterization scheduled for this afternoon. I know he must be starving by now, but so am I. There are several Indian dishes, all so delicious I try to eat every bite—the beginning of a bad habit. Howard rests, and I eat some of the best Indian food I've ever put in my mouth.

Soon, he sits up and says, "I think I finally identified the feeling I had during our last days at home."

I am eager to hear this, because I've assumed he has put feelings of any kind on a back burner. I put down my fork. "Tell me."

He looks a bit wistful and says, "It was like driving around on a tank of gas without a gas gauge, having no idea how much longer before I ran out of gas and the car stopped."

I want to applaud his insight, but I nod instead. "I'm sure you had plenty of gas or Dr. Engel would have admitted you immediately," I say. "But I understand exactly what you mean." I recall my frustration with his wanting to finish the kitchen renovation job he was working on before coming here. There is some comfort in knowing he is starting to grasp the significance of his diagnosis.

"I think I didn't want to admit it," Howard says.

"Well, we're here now, and you're getting it taken care of," I say. "You're in good hands now."

A young man knocks and enters. He wears a gray wrap-around jacket and such an enormous smile that I can only smile back at him. He motions for Howard to follow him. It is only when Howard returns that I find out he has gone to the "treatment room" to be shaved—prep for the catheterization.

"He shaved me dry!" Howard says, pointing to his belly and groin. "A straight razor and quick!" He makes slashing motions in the air. "Zip. Zap. Zip. Done! Like Zorro."

Sheela comes in with another wheelchair. "Mr. Howard must go to Cath Lab now," she says. "We bring him back soon."

"May I come, too?" I ask.

"No, we bring him to you. It is not long."

Now they will stick a catheter through an artery in Howard's groin.

Dr. Engel had explained that they would do a catheterization to check for any blockages in his arteries, so if there are any, they can take care of them during the valve surgery. Sheela hands the wheelchair to a young man and turns to Howard. "Come," she says, and helps him into his seat. I pray a silent prayer that he won't say, "I don't need help!"

I lean down to kiss Howard good-bye. "Come home soon," I say, without any idea at all of how much like home this room will become for me.

When Howard returns to the room after his catheterization, he is on a stretcher. His eyes are sparkling and he stretches his neck to crow like a rooster. "I have not only good, but excellent arteries!" he announces. "No blockages! I can eat all the chocolate I want."

"They never said that," I say.

Three sisters transfer him into his bed. First he was walking, then in a wheelchair, then a stretcher, and now in his hospital bed, instructed not to move—a sequence that feels like visual preparation for the shock of what looms in the future—something that was once quite distant and blurred, that now is zooming into view.

"Now you eat lunch," one nurse says to Howard. She explains that Howard must stay in bed for six hours, and his left leg must be kept flat with a "sandbag" weighting down the artery's entrance site. The pressure on his artery and bladder during the procedure makes him need to pee badly, so we get our first experience with bedpans. After several successful attempts, he devours his very own Indian non-vegetarian ("non-veg") meal complete with a fruit plate of pomegranate, papaya, apples, and pears.

"This is better Indian food than we ever get back home," he says.

"I know," I say. "If I keep eating all they give me, I'll need to buy an extra seat for our return flight."

In very short order, Howard is visited by Dr. Gupta, a cardiothoracic surgeon. With each additional doctor we meet, I become more acutely aware that we have not yet seen Dr. Trehan. I resign myself to the possibility that Dr. Trehan may not even do the surgery, he has so many assistants. But that doesn't frighten or even frustrate me. These doctors and nurses are so competent, so thorough, and so prompt, that my confidence builds with each interaction, with each test.

Dr. Gupta takes another complete medical history, and then asks Howard about his stuttering. "Did your speech problem begin with your heart symptoms?"

"No," Howard says, "at about age four, when I began to t-t-t-t-t-t-t-t-t ... talk." Being the youngest of three children, his siblings probably spoke for him, or he was simply given what he needed and not encouraged to ask for things.

Since I met Howard, he has been teaching me what he's learned about stuttering; about the familial pattern of stutterers creating stutterers. Although most parents know that repetition is the most basic and natural part of learning to speak, stuttering parents, out of fear that their children will also stutter, try to prevent their children from repeating words. "Say it only once!" his parents used to yell at him. "Do not repeat!" What a sad legacy to give a child.

Dr. Gupta nods. "You will be seen by a neurologist, urologist, and we will schedule your surgery within one or two days." This is Saturday, so I calculate Monday, confirming what Dr. K. said earlier. "Your TEE suggests that the valve can be repaired," Dr. Gupta says, as if this news is an afterthought. "We will try. But this can only be determined at the time of surgery. If we cannot repair it, we will replace it." Great news!

A technician rolls an ECG (electrocardiogram) analyzer into the room, as if on cue, and Dr. Gupta continues, "You will be connected to this monitoring machine." As he speaks, he attaches five leads to Howard's heart. "But you must not move your leg for six more hours."

About thirty minutes later, Naruna (one of the fellows who met us at the airport) calls our room to say Dr. Trehan is getting out of surgery now, and is sending for us.

"But Howard cannot move his leg for six hours," I say.

"I will come there," Naruna says quickly. He hangs up.

I am instantly struck by two facts: first, that Dr. Trehan is actually here and doing surgery on a Saturday, and second, that he is sending for Howard instead of coming to see him in his room.

Naruna comes to our room, and I explain again that Howard is not supposed to get up until 8:30 P.M. because of the catheterization and the need to keep his leg still and weighted by the sandbag. "I will come back," Naruna says.

In the next couple of hours, the urologist comes, Sanjiv brings me a map and guidebook of Delhi, and a man with a turban comes to greet us and ask if we need anything— anything at all. I explain that I would like to know where I can find an Internet café, so I can e-mail home. He takes me down to the nurses' station and tells me to use the computer there anytime. It seems like such an intrusion that I shake my head, and say, "I don't want to disturb the nurses. I must e-mail our family often."

He insists it is no problem and tells the head nurse, "Sister Deepti, she is to use the computer anytime."

"Of course." The nurses scurry about, clearing counter space, moving chairs, making way for me to enter their workstation.

I am embarrassed. "No, no, not now," I say, waving my hands to stop their packing up. "Thank you. I will come back. Thank you very much." I must try to assess the low-traffic times before I invade a station that buzzes with nurses and doctors. But I am anxious to try out the system we set up before we left. I e-mail Jackie, and Jackie posts the progress report on www.howardsheart.com, so that anyone, anywhere can read what's going on. Our families and Howard's friends are all over the world, and I was grateful for Jackie's offer to handle the Web site while we are gone.

I return to our room and to Howard, high in his bed, fast asleep, the familiar whistling of air from between his lips. What a day it has been, and we still have not met the man we will trust to hold Howard's heart in his hands and mend those delicate heartstrings.

While Howard sleeps, I look out the window where the background of our drama is as commonplace to the people in the street as it is mysterious to us. Bicyclists balance 14- or 16-foot bamboo ladders on their shoulders. Workers with long scarves draped down their backs pedal wagon rickshaws loaded with tall rolls of sheet metal or a few steel pipes. Trucks pass with workers sitting atop the load of debris. Men walk by, some stopping to pee at the jog (a 90-degree angle) in the long gray wall.

The next knock at the door brings the Senior Manager of Finance. Howard sleeps through our discussion about payment. I tell him we haven't changed enough money into Indian currency yet, prepared to explain about our arrival and all that has happened since.

"Do you have credit card?" he asks me.

"Yes, of course." I find the credit card and reluctantly leave Howard to follow this man to pay. All the way to the basement I worry about how I will be able to tell how much I am paying, how to be sure I will understand what is covered. I know the currency here is called "rupees" but have no idea what the exchange rate for U.S. dollars is in rupees.

"You just pay five thousand U.S. dollars today," the finance man explains. I stand at the small teller window ready to exchange a swipe of our MasterCard for Howard's repaired heart.

When I return to the room, instead of finding Howard asleep, there is a team of several doctors and sisters circling Howard's bed. I can almost hear my heart, it is beating so wildly, wondering what could have happened while I was gone. They break the circle and make a path for me, when I recognize Dr. Trehan from his picture on the Escorts Web site. He stands beside Howard. We shake hands and he resumes talking about their strategy.

"It looks as if we will be able to repair the valve," he says to me, "and if not, we will replace it." I nod, and say a silent prayer that the repair is possible.

A crazy thought flashes across my mind—a friend facing a mastectomy who had opted to have both breasts removed "while they were at it," so she would never have to worry again. I wonder if there is any benefit to just starting over with a brand-new valve.

"Is there any reason to just go ahead and replace it?" I ask.

Dr. Trehan looks a bit surprised, then seems to understand. "It is always better to keep your own body part if possible," he says. I nod. "But if we determine that a successful repair is not possible, we will be prepared to replace it with a new valve." I am relieved at his patience and at how much sense this all makes so far. His English is impeccable. He continues, "The catheterization shows no stenosis, no blockage in any arteries."

"So I can eat all the chocolate I want," Howard interjects.

More sideways glances then laughter around the circle, and Dr. Trehan continues. "The results of all the other tests should be back by Monday morning, so we will schedule the surgery for Monday afternoon." He discusses the choice between the tissue valve ("pig valve," as Howard calls it) and the metal "St. Jude" valve. Dr. Trehan explains the choice almost identically to the way Dr. Engel had described it.

The St. Jude valve lasts much longer, but necessitates that Howard be on blood thinners for the rest of his life. In Howard's construction business, should he suffer even a minor cut on the job, or a scraped knee from bike riding, there would be a high risk of not being able to stop the bleeding. The pig valve lasts only ten to fifteen years, but requires no blood thinner. Dr. Engel said the choice was up to Howard.

"In ten years, they will have perfected some simple laser surgery to put in a new valve," Howard says. "Something noninvasive, and quick, just like that!" He snaps his fingers.

"Perhaps," says Dr. Trehan. "It is your choice. But in your line of work...."

"I choose the pig valve," Howard says, as if announcing a verdict. I am grateful he does not look to me to help him decide.

Dr. Trehan nods in approval. "A reasonable decision." I look around to detect any dissension among the team, but everyone seems content. "Tonight you eat a good meal," Dr. Trehan continues, "and we will get a Doppler of your leg. Tomorrow you rest."

Tomorrow is Sunday, and Howard must be thinking what I am thinking. "May we go out to see some of the city tomorrow?" he asks.

Quick looks around the circle, then everyone's eyes rest on Dr. Trehan to answer. "No, it is best if you stay inside. We do not want to risk anything from the outside." Howard and I do not understand the scope of this risk, but before we can ask, Dr. Trehan says, "You are in somewhat of a controlled environment here. Wait until after the surgery." He turns to me, "How long do you plan to stay in India?"

"Our return tickets are for one month," I say, "but they can be changed if we need to."

He shakes his head. "Not necessary. That is perfect. You will have plenty of time to sightsee."

When the team leaves, it is already time to put in our dinner order. I decide to stick with Indian veg, and Howard orders Indian non-veg. "Do you have any chocolate?" he adds.

From the look on the dietitian woman's face, he might as well have asked for double whiskey. Then she smiles, most likely deciding it is a joke. "Not at Escorts," she says, and puts her pen in her pocket. She repeats Howard's order and all that will come with his chicken.

"And a candy bar," Howard says. "Anything chocolate. Please."

"I ask for you," she promises before she leaves.

"Howard, something tells me the only chocolate to be found here might be in someone's desk drawer," I say. "This is, after all, a hospital full of heart patients."

"But I have perfectly clear arteries," he argues. "I've been eating chocolate for fifty-three years and have not just good but excellent arteries!"

"I'll go outside and buy you a candy bar," I say. "I'll smuggle it in if I have to."

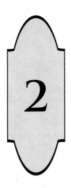

2

What's a Healthy Guy Like You Doing in a Place Like This?

Sunday, September 26, 2004

Sunday is our day of rest, which neither Howard nor I do well if we are unable to venture outdoors. We do leave our room, though, and walk the hallways on the fourth floor from one guard to the next. We stop at every window to look at Delhi from any angle possible.

Occasionally, a guard will point to a building in the distance and say, "Lotus Temple" or "hospital" or "mosque"—nouns they have learned to say in English. Then back to our room for the crossword puzzles I tear out of every English-version newspaper that arrives with breakfast or that I find in the hallway. We read the books we brought with us—poetry, novels.

Each time someone from food service comes in with tea or a dietitian comes to take Howard's meal order, Howard asks, "Did you find any chocolate yet?" I start to feel sorry for these employees who obviously have nothing to do with chocolate bars.

By late afternoon, I am torn between not wanting to leave Howard and feeling stir-crazy from only watching the sunny day, instead of feeling sun on my face. We agree I will go outside and look for colored markers or pencils or crayons, some paper to draw on, and yes ... a chocolate bar.

I must go down in an elevator and find my way outside the hospital for the first time, then cross the busy street I have watched from four floors up. Howard promises to wave to me from our window.

Outside, I feel like Steve McQueen in *The Great Escape*. I make it past uniformed guards at every elevator and every door. They all wave me on, even the one at the guardhouse by the big wrought iron gate that separates the dust and chaos of New Delhi from our pristine world inside Escorts. I get the sense that someone has pinned a huge sign on my back that says "American," then realize it hardly would be necessary. Still, it is disconcerting to imagine Dr. Trehan informing all of these doctors, sisters, and security guards about Howard and me coming to their hospital.

I walk down the middle of the street lined with the vendors' carts I saw from our room, and know I am going the right way. I look up and spot Howard. He is standing in the window, shirtless, the white leads from his "pocket heart monitor" are stuck to his chest. From here, he looks as if someone has drawn a road map on his chest with the white wires.

He waves. I wave back, then feel self-conscious when passersby smile at me. I decide there is no way to be inconspicuous on this street, and I'll be better off watching where I step, so I don't run into a rickshaw or trip over a dog. I get nervous at the far edge of the Escorts property when I can no longer see the patient rooms, and I turn back. I haven't found any shops yet, but I remember that from some view on the fourth floor, I saw cell phone stores and a sign that said "Chemist," which I'd assumed was a pharmacy.

I enter a busy intersection to cross to the opposite side of the street, buses and cars, bicycles, and the little green auto-rickshaws all honking and zigzagging in front of and behind me. I decide to just go for it, and land safely on the other side. But the other side isn't really designated by sidewalks or safe pedestrian-only areas. It's sort of a free-for-all, like booths at a flea market spilling into each other and then into the roadway.

I find an open storefront that carries an odd assortment of magazines, pads of paper, candy. I point to the paper, and then enlarge some imaginary framed space in midair with my hands to indicate "big paper." The boy goes to the back of the stall and points to a piece of paper. "Bigger?" I ask. I end up with a couple of large sheets of paper—a little dusty, but blank—and a small set of colored markers. Then I see the Kit Kat candy bars in a box. Howard loves dark chocolate, but I figure he'll take what he gets. I ask about wine or beer.

After several clerks try to figure out what I am saying, another customer translates. Everyone giggles, but I am too ignorant to be embarrassed. When they begin pointing down the street and shouting directions in Hindi, I realize this is not going to be easy. The sun feels good on my skin, so I wander a bit more, feeling quite brave. I try to relax, walk as though I've been here before and know when to jump over garbage and water. I watch a young boy sewing layers of batting for a comforter spread out on the ground. I pass a store that displays white hospital clothes like Howard's new karate uniform, a photocopy store, but nothing that looks like wine or beer.

I head back to the hospital struck by some irrational fear that I won't be allowed back in, that I will be stuck out here, without Howard. Crazy thoughts run through my head like, "They've got Howard and five thousand dollars from the MasterCard ... what do they need me for?" I dodge cars and bicycles, and pretend not to hear the vendors calling to me.

As I make my way back, I think of what a difference a couple of days make. Time has been balled up and dried out like one of those compressed washcloths that fits inside a plastic egg—add water, and it springs back to normal wash-cloth size. I try to remember back to when the subject of Howard's heart did not exist in our world, way before we ever spoke the words "India," "New Delhi," or even "surgery." But I can only reach back as far as last Thursday, when we left North Carolina.

Thursday, September 23, 2004

On the afternoon of our departure for India, we could have just as easily been heading to Atlanta or New York City for a weekend. Our friend Sarina had arrived at my house at 2:00 P.M. After some casual conversation about our kids, we loaded up our bags (which we'd wisely kept to one each), and drove toward the Raleigh-Durham airport. Howard wanted to stop to buy a portable CD player, so Sarina pulled into the new Southpoint mall just off I-40. While Howard shopped, Sarina bought a tuna sandwich at Panera Bread. I sat in the car. I doubt that anyone was thinking about India. It wouldn't become a real part of our thoughts for some time.

Now, I know that nothing could have prepared us for anything that remotely resembled the journey we were about to make. Sarina dropped us at the curb outside the American Airlines terminal. We hugged her, thanked her, and said, "See you in one month."

We hadn't thought about our tickets since we authorized our travel agent, Sally, to book them, but we found ourselves in front of a self-serve, check-in machine that resembled a slot machine more than anything to do with air travel. A ticket agent helped us when she realized we were just staring at the screen. We were caught off guard when she handed us our tickets and boarding passes and said, "Your bags are checked all the way to Delhi." She looked at Howard. "If you'll sit over there, your wheelchair is on its way."

Even in my surprise, I was sure that I'd detected a slight roll of her eyes. After all, he was obviously not crippled, and didn't even look sick. We had both forgotten that our travel agent had requested wheelchair assistance for Howard on all connections because she didn't want Howard to have to run to meet any flight.

Soon, our first attendant arrived with a wheelchair. Her gray, disheveled hair and airport pallor, I assumed, echoed her level of interest in her job. She took our tickets. Howard climbed in and insisted on holding both of our backpacks in his lap. By the playful light in his eyes, I knew he wanted to wheel himself, race me down the terminal, and pop a wheelie somewhere. Luckily, the attendant seemed to be all business.

I walked alongside empty-handed as she wove in and out of passengers, bypassed the long lines, and got us through Security without having to wait. About halfway to our gate, she said, "I know where you're going." Howard and I swapped glances. "Saw you on the six o'clock news last night."

We'd heard from friends that our story had been repeated on various broadcasts since our first TV interview with Tim Nelson of Channel 11, ABC *Eyewitness News*.

The gray-haired woman pushed Howard up to a very crowded gate, jockeyed his wheelchair around to park next to the only empty seat, and motioned for me to sit down. She patted Howard on the shoulder and whispered, "Good luck to you over there."

Luck hadn't entered my mind, and it seemed an odd sentiment—as if things could go badly.

The eighty-something woman I sat beside in the gate area asked if we were headed to Detroit. We both shook our heads. I answered, "India." After a brief exchange of travel plans, she told us of a magazine article she'd just read about all the claims America makes for being top dog. "In my opinion," she said, "the U.S. is number one in only one way." She hoped we would guess. "America is the country the rest of the world fears the most."

I was reminded of the first interview we did a couple of weeks ago with the *Chapel Hill Herald* reporter. At that interview, Howard had said, "I think the insurance companies are the true terrorists in our country, causing everyone to live in fear of disaster." I knew the second he said it that it would become the italicized pull-out quote the editor would enlarge and set in its own little box in the center of the page. And it was. I hoped it wouldn't haunt us.

When we landed in Detroit, the attendant who met us with a wheelchair was responsible for getting us to our connecting gate before they closed the doors. We kept tally of our gratitude to Sally for having had the foresight to arrange for this assistance. People, especially business passengers, must spend more time on Jetways than they do on freeways. But it had been a while since either of us had flown beyond the shores of the U.S.

After we found our seats on the next flight to Amsterdam, I asked to speak to the head flight attendant. "I am the Purser," she corrected me. I explained why we were flying to India, thinking someone besides me should be aware of Howard's medical condition in case he started coughing or . . . worse. The Purser was unruffled by the news. "That's okay. I'm also a nurse," she said, and repeated our seat numbers out loud.

I noticed that all the passengers had a movie screen suspended directly in front of their seats. I was impressed. No more craning my neck to see around the sea of heads between me and the movie screen mounted on those carpeted partitions between first and coach class.

What I found nearly as intriguing were the monitors hanging over the aisles, showing our plane's location during the flight. It was a sort of follow-the-bouncing-ball-over-song-lyrics idea, where a tiny red icon of a plane hovered over colorful continents and large expanses of water, moving as we traveled at 600 miles per hour. Just as on MapQuest, the map shifted to include more of what lay east and south of us as we approached new territory on our route. Seeing the Netherlands and Scandinavia come into view was interesting, and new; I'd never been that far north in Europe before.

The copilot announced that the flight would be a little over seven hours. The featured movie was *Garfield*. My flu symptoms caused by the malaria pills were finally dissipating, but I suddenly remembered the dream I'd had the night before of being lost in a hospital, sleeping on wet gravel, and being unable to locate Dr. Trehan. I was looking forward to sleep. I found *Dirty Dancing: Havana Nights* on a different channel and watched that instead of *Garfield* before a nap and our rainy descent into Amsterdam, an orderly patchwork of canals and greenhouses.

On the final flight from Amsterdam to New Delhi, the tiny red plane left a wake of its flight path on the overhead monitor, reminding me of watching close-ups of Coach K drawing a last minute three-point maneuver for the Duke Blue Devils. (Mike Krzyzewski, Duke University's basketball coach, is called Coach K by college basketball fans.) The names of cities became not only unfamiliar, but unpronounceable, much like Howard's diagnosis had seemed in the beginning: "Flailing mitral valve with prolapse and severe regurgitation." I watched the little red plane icon fly over Germany, Poland, the Ukraine, Russia, Iran, and Afghanistan. My throat tightened.

We saw Tehran. Then the tip of our plane pointed to Kabul.

"Howard, look. I haven't seen Kabul on a map since the CNN coverage of the war."

"Well, why would we?" he says. "It's like Iraq. Who keeps a map of Iraq in their glove compartment?"

"We're really going to India," I said, and took his hand. My astonished realization might have been a normal part of our pretravel preparations, had I not succumbed to the too-busy-to-register syndrome (or was it simple denial?). And the phenomenon is not new to me.

Thirty years ago, I spent a month living with my older sister in her college apartment. Because she was living so far from our parents, I helped with all of her wedding arrangements. I was so busy, so consumed with my many tasks, that the impact of her getting married didn't hit me until I walked down the aisle ahead of her. I saw the harpist we had hired and began to cry. I never heard the vows they had written, never heard the songs people sang. I couldn't stop crying until after the reception that night.

"I don't even know where India is!" I tell Howard who still has his eyes closed.

"It's over by Africa," he says, still a bit on the nap side of my discovery.

And that seems the extent of what we know about India, even though the last two weeks have been packed full of plans to spend at least the next month over there.

Not until some time between supper and breakfast, two of the best airplane meals I ever had—Indian vegetarian (curry turnovers, pistachio ice cream, wine, and Heineken)— did Howard pull out the copies of Dr. Engel's medical notes we were to hand-deliver to Dr. Trehan. Thinking we would read the same haunting diagnosis and the long names for all the presurgery procedures Howard would now have done in India instead of Durham, I watched over his shoulder. He leafed through test results and handwritten notes.

"Get this," he said, pointing to an embedded paragraph halfway down.

I read aloud, "Patient insists he is asymptomatic ..." and a bit farther down, "We are amazed that this patient is not already in heart failure."

Howard looked at me, as if I had been keeping this secret from him.

"Guess it's better we didn't hear that before now," I said, trying not to let the urgency register on my face. "We wouldn't have done anything differently."

I thought to myself, rather smugly, about the night we'd both lost it, the one and only time. We had seen Dr. Engel for Howard's last visit, picked up copies of his medical records, and later that evening, talked about what day to leave for India. Howard had suggested going in a couple of weeks.

He and his crew were renovating an old house. "If we can just finish the kitchen, then Rachel can move in the day she closes on her other house. The screened porch can wait till I get back."

"Howard! Did you hear what you just said?" My reaction was sharply bristled, I'm sure, by the fact that this current renovation job was for his ex-girlfriend. "Forget Rachel's kitchen! I don't care if she sleeps in her car and eats at McDonalds while we're gone. This is your heart we're talking about, Howard!"

The argument went on like that for a while:

"What's a couple of more weeks?"

"It could mean your life!"

"I promised her we'd meet the moving day deadline."

"Anyone else would understand this change in plans."

"But I don't have to change it."

"How selfish can Rachel be?"

Finally, I realized that Rachel had not even been approached about the need to change plans. Howard was procrastinating. Dropping everything and hopping on a plane to India added drama and reality to a situation we still hadn't truly come to grips with. But it was time to do exactly that. Howard's sixteen-year-old son, Alan, even chimed in, "Dad, just go! The sooner you go, the sooner you'll be back."

By the following afternoon, Howard had found a long-time friend and fellow builder to step in and oversee the renovations. Rachel was perfectly fine with the crew continuing without Howard. He left his crew detailed instructions of how to complete the work. And, as with so many seemingly insignificant turns of event, Howard's departure was an unforeseen gift to his crew's foreman—for the first time, he got to step up to the plate and truly take charge.

Back in June, Howard had bought his first new bicycle. About the same time, some subconscious trigger reminded him that he hadn't had a routine physical for quite sometime, so he called his doctor to schedule an appointment. Two weeks later, while she palpated his neck and looked in his ears and eyes, Howard and his doctor, a former customer of his, caught up. They talked about their kids, about this year's Merle Fest music festival they always attended together, about what her husband was up to. Then she pulled out her stethoscope from her coat's deep pocket and gave his heart a listen.

Howard was finishing a sentence which, since he stutters, can sometimes take a while.

"Shhhh!" his doctor interrupted him. She listened again. "Oh my!" She knew the murmur in his heart was a new sound, never detected before that day's examination. Howard called me after the appointment and said, "Guess what? I have a heart murmur."

I swallowed. "My sister had a heart murmur thirty years ago; lots of people have heart murmurs."

"She seemed pretty surprised," Howard said. "I told her I'd get it checked out when we get back." We were scheduled to leave for a two-week trip to Nova Scotia in a few days, a trip we had been looking forward to for months. "She said I needed to have an echocardiogram immediately."

"You mean before we go?" I asked. I remember thinking, "There's nothing like going to a doctor for a routine checkup to suddenly find out you're sick."

I went with Howard to the lab at Duke University first thing in the morning. The next day, his doctor called him with the diagnosis: a flailing mitral valve with prolapse. I looked it up online, read about all the patients who have mitral valve prolapse and who take medicine for many years to control it. His doctor said we could go on our trip, but that we had to see a cardiologist as soon as we got back.

We relaxed—a little. We went on the trip. Part of it involved reinforcing a friend's cabin that was rotting out and collapsing on the side of a Cape Breton mountain. Howard jacked up the cabin and replaced some rotten posts. We crawled around under the main house, dragged out rotted wood, and installed a fan and vents to combat the moisture problem. We got in a few short hikes, camped by a lake during the tail end of Hurricane Alex, and walked all over Halifax, where we dried out before our trip home.

When we returned, we saw Dr. Engel, the cardiologist who had been recommended to us by every person I asked, including Howard's primary care physician who first heard Howard's heart murmur. Dr. Engel reviewed the diagnosis from his echocardiogram, which suddenly had grown in length: "Hypercontractile left ventricle function with mild LVH. Valvular regurgitation; trivial AR, severe MR. No valvular stenosis. Posterior MVP with partially flailing posterior MV leaflet. Severe mitral regurgitation. Morphology: prolapse"; in short, "a flailing mitral valve with prolapse and severe mitral regurgitation."

Apparently, the Duke technician who'd called Howard's doctor with the results of his echocardiogram a few weeks ago had read only part of the diagnosis. Dr. Engel was clear and precise, and immediately won our complete confidence. She examined Howard and listened intently. Then, she held out the stethoscope's earpieces for each of us to listen to his heart. "Hear that whooshing noise?" she asked. It was like the sound of someone swishing a towel back and forth through water. Yes, we heard it.

Dr. Engel described the heart's valves as being like the two halves of a parachute that must fill, then collapse, then fill again, held taut by strings. Howard's "anchor strings" had snapped. "Suddenly," she said, "and no one knows why." She left very little cause for doubt. I told her about what I'd read online about mitral valve prolapse. She confirmed that people with mitral valve prolapse (bulging) or stenosis (blockage) often take medication and live normal lives for many years, as long as they are carefully watched by their cardiologists.

"But Howard's case is so severe," she said, "that it will require surgery as soon as possible, either to repair or replace the mitral valve. That's the flailing part." She looked directly into both of our eyes to emphasize the difference. "The severe regurgitation means the blood is backing up, without the valve to keep it in the heart."

Looking back, our next confession was the fulcrum on which our story turned: "Howard has no health insurance," I said.

Dr. Engel looked horrified, then she quickly changed her expression to a noncommittal one. Because I had administered employee benefits in several previous jobs, I knew all about pre-existing conditions. "If we get him insurance now," I said, "it will be a year before they will cover any problem connected with his heart, I'm sure. Can it wait that long?"

Dr. Engel took a deep breath. "No." The room was silent for one of those distorted moments that seems to stretch into an enormous span of time. "Howard cannot wait a year for his surgery." She looked at me. "Maggi, you are going to have to be assertive. Make an appointment with the CFO of the hospital and see if you can work out a payment plan. Howard, this is not just going to set you back financially, this will be staggering."

At that moment, I took charge. I called Durham Regional Hospital and asked for the names of the CEO, the CFO, and for their phone numbers. The operator connected me with the CFO's secretary. I explained that I wanted to make an appointment with the CFO, and she suggested two o'clock the next afternoon. I'd been expecting the royal runaround, so I fumbled for a minute, then accepted, and told her our names.

The next day Howard and I met Mr. Craig Damien, the CFO, who had invited two other patient financial personnel to join us. The five of us sat around a table. Grateful for the appointment in the first place, I wanted to take as little of their time as possible. Howard and I had agreed that it would be best if I explained the story. I can talk much faster than Howard, whose stutter can become pronounced when he is put on the spot.

I thanked them all for taking the time to meet with us and explained the situation: "Howard is a self-employed, fifty-three-year-old carpenter, and the single parent of a sixteen-year-old son. He is a person who prides himself on meeting deadlines and sticking to the financial estimates that he promises his customers. He has volunteered as a carpenter with Habitat for Humanity."

All eyes on me, I kept going, wanting to give an accurate picture of Howard as an honest, pay-as-you-go kind of guy, not wanting a handout. "Howard is a nonsmoker; he prepares meals for himself and his son with vegetables from their own garden; he forbids sodas, junk food, and TV in his home. And he makes sure that he and his son go for regular physical and dental checkups. Howard has paid out-of-pocket for every medical visit, and every prescription he's ever needed, for his whole life. He has even been known to pay for a friend's medical or dental emergency treatment simply because Howard could, and the friend could not.

"Howard has been healthy," I said, "until now." I explained the sudden diagnosis and Dr. Engel's recommendation for surgery as soon as possible. And then, the bottom line: "Howard has no health insurance," I said.

There was a woman at the meeting whose job it was to help patients apply for Medicaid. But Howard and I both knew that he would never qualify for Medicaid. "He is not indigent. He makes a decent living and pays his bills on time," I explained.

"So we would like to get an estimate for the cost of everything—the surgery, the operating room, the anesthesiologist—everything," I said. "But we are here to ask you to please accept what an insurance company would pay you for this surgery."

The three of them looked at each other. The CFO spoke. "We have no way to do that."

From my years of billing insurance companies for patients' surgery, I knew that hospitals and doctors must agree to accept whatever the insurance companies deem the "usual and customary fee" for any given procedure. I also knew the medical provider often writes off any remaining balance unless a patient has a secondary insurance.

"But Mr. Damien, the self-pay patient faces the total charges, which are arbitrary amounts set by the provider." No one moved. I kept going. "We would like to offer to pay you the same amount that any insurance company would pay, so you won't be out anything." Silence. "We can pay you a substantial amount up front, I'm sure. Then we have plans to raise enough money to pay the rest as soon as possible."

I explained our idea of a party, with bands, dancing, food, kegs of beer, maybe even an art auction. "You are all invited." They smiled the kind of stick-on, peel-off smiles they are paid to carry in their pockets.

Mr. Damien looked at his Financial Advisor. "Do you know what the hospital bill might be for mitral valve surgery?"

Mr. Finance shuffled in his seat and mumbled about how he could find out later, how the procedure usually entailed a five-to-seven-day stay, hmmmm....

"Just a ballpark figure," the CFO urged him.

Mr. Finance fidgeted a bit longer, then mumbled, "Close to $100,000." Then he looked up at Howard with newly resurrected confidence. "And we would need half up front, the rest on a payment plan," he said as if we were buying a new dishwasher from Sears.

The CFO reviewed. "$100,000. And that is just for the hospital bill, five to seven days, right?" he said.

Mr. Finance nodded.

"That is, if there are no complications," the CFO said, and then turned to Howard. "And the surgeon, cardiologist, anesthesiologist, radiologist, pathologist, the valve itself, and any medications prescribed will all be billed separately."

Howard nodded. "I understand."

"That $100,000 includes the operating room and the hospital room for five to seven days, right?" I asked.

"Yes. But everything else is separate, and you'd have to ask each of them what their bills will be." Mr. Finance took over the conversation from Mr. Damien. "And the surgeon will probably want half up front too. And if the stay is longer, the cost would increase."

"Yes, and I'm asking what an insurance company, like mine—Blue Cross Blue Shield—would pay you for that $100,000 hospital bill."

The air in the room thickened. All three of them were squirming. I was sure my neck was getting blotchy the way it did in my wedding pictures, or any other time I got flustered.

"We are not set up to compromise that way," said the CFO.

I looked directly at him. "Mr. Damien, surely we are not the only self-pay patients who face surgery this costly."

"No." he said. He paused a long time before he spoke again. "No, but you are the first to come to us ahead of time to talk about it."

I was stunned. "What do the others do?"

Mr. Finance spoke up. "They usually come in an ambulance to the Emergency Room, and then we talk about payment later."

The woman added, "And we help them apply to Medicaid."

"And you end up writing off bad debts," I said. I shifted to sit up taller in my seat. "Look, we want to pay you. And we don't want to wait until Howard has to come in an ambulance. I'm asking you to work with us so we can pay you every cent you would get if Howard was an insured patient."

Mr. Damien looked at his lap as if he'd dropped his cue card. Then he turned to me and repeated, "We just aren't set up for that."

The meeting was over and we were on our way with applications they insisted we take with us—applications that asked for Howard's tax returns, his W-2s, and other financial information that would disqualify him immediately. Mr. Finance promised to call the next day with a more exact estimate of the hospital charges.

And call he did. He had done his research, and the official estimate was $98,000, if there were no complications. We could probably count on all the other medical bills doubling that figure. Our new estimate was now a staggering $200,000, if there were no complications, an additional phrase that unnerved me each time someone added it to the end of his or her sentence.

Ironically, my best friend's mother had been admitted to this very hospital two months before, for a valve replacement. She was in the cardiac intensive care unit for weeks before she stabilized enough to be moved to a private room upstairs. Her stay, originally estimated at the same five-to-seven days, grew into a thirty-eight-day marathon. I wondered what her complications had cost, and how much more they would cost an uninsured patient.

Howard went to work. I began looking into health insurance for him. I got the names of brokers from friends who had miraculously obtained insurance for their children after severe accidents. I would even have purchased "disaster insurance," as policies with very high deductibles are called. Even if Howard had to pay the first $5,000 up front, any insurance policy could help.

I applied to AARP for insurance for Howard. I called my own insurance agent to ask what Howard's premium would be with Blue Cross Blue Shield of North Carolina. He faxed us a quote for a policy that cost over $300 a month based on his age and history. Then I told him about the mitral valve diagnosis. He assured me they could cover him, but warned me that the premiums would most likely go up to cover the additional risk. The new quote was over $1,600 a month. The policy would disallow any claims related to his heart diagnosis for a year or longer since it was now a pre-existing condition. We did the math. Sixteen hundred dollars a month for twelve months equaled almost $20,000 a year, with no assistance for the surgery he needed now. I began to plan the fund-raiser.

I had been to countless benefits. I'd bought several "plate dinners" to raise funds for other people's medical needs. I had donated many pieces of my artwork to auctions designed to raise money for victims of autism and cancer. Friends suggested a golf tournament, a bike ride, a "pig pickin'" ... all to raise funds to help with hospital bills.

It was September, still plenty of long sunny days and warm nights. We decided to have a party. We would call it "Howard's Hoe-Down" and hold it in Howard's barn. Howard knew folks in the food business. My younger son, Thane, and I knew a lot of local musicians. But the musicians had to be paid. The caterers had to at least cover their real costs, they couldn't just donate food. As an artist, I'd been asked to donate my time and artwork far more often than I was asked to sell it.

Howard had been asked to repair friends' houses or to help build Habitat homes more times than he could remember. Neither of us wanted to take advantage of our friends who might earn even less money than Howard did. We were advised and were finally convinced that the Hoe-Down would not be effective and it would be a lot of hard work to pull off. But where were we going to scrounge $200,000? Or even "half up front"? Sell our homes?

Friends pulled together. One wrote a letter that we mailed to friends and former customers of Howard's, all of whom loved him. We wanted to inform everyone of the situation that would undoubtedly take Howard out of the normal work loop for some months, and also to offer suggestions to answer the inevitable and recurring question, "How can we help?"

Financial contributions were only one need, and we also sought understanding and prayers, perhaps transportation for Howard's son when Howard was in the hospital, and food—people always need meals prepared for the family following surgery. I opened a new bank account called "Howard's Heart." A new sense of urgency took over.

Rather quickly, I began to recognize this as a broader political issue than simply Howard's predicament alone. Public awareness edged its way into my list of priorities, and I replayed the chant I had heard so many writers use for so many years: "the personal is the political." We sent the same letter of explanation via countless e-mails to even more distant relatives. I sent press releases to local journalists, hoping someone might pick up Howard's story as a human interest piece.

Tactfully, friends helped spread the word. One wrote to Oprah. Another called a news reporter she'd never met, but whose writing she admired. Our good friend Sarina told a woman she worked out with at her gym about our situation, which led to our first television interview. The press began calling. I handled the calls because Howard was still trying to work as much as he could. He was more fatigued than either of us admitted. And although he is quite articulate, there was the added effort it takes for anyone who stutters to speak fluently and publicly.

Reactions to Howard's news ranged from "He was irresponsible not to have health insurance in the first place," to "This kind of thing has been my worst nightmare.... I also have no health insurance by choice," to "I can't even afford health insurance for my children, let alone myself." Donations dribbled in. We felt slightly guilty when we saw each personal check. But I reminded Howard that he had written many checks to help others. It was his turn to learn how to accept help, and simply say thank you.

From my research we learned that Howard was not the only one who, though apparently healthy and physically fit, would face surprising news of this kind without health insurance in place. In fact, he was only one of about forty-six million Americans who remain uninsured, either by necessity or by choice. (Between 16 and 17 percent of North Carolinians had been uninsured over the previous three years.)

My older son, Bryan, sent an e-mail one afternoon that gave this formless chaos a new center. He had traveled to India the summer after his first year of medical school at Stanford. His anatomy professor, Dr. Srivastava, had set him up with a three-week rotation at one of the public hospitals in New Delhi. Bryan had just returned to California the week we got the "staggering figure" from the Durham hospital, and after our friends had discouraged us from having the Howard's Hoe-Down fund-raiser. It was Bryan who'd first suggested India:

> Dear Mom, I'll e-mail some people and ask about various international options. In the meantime, here are some Web sites and info on the Apollo Hospitals, which I visited—the Delhi branch. It is a private hospital, an absolutely beautiful, pristine facility, with standards every bit as high as most American hospitals (at least as far as this not-yet-health-care-professional can tell). The chain is based in Chennai in the south of India—(aka Madras) but they have hospitals all over India. They actively recruit this sort of business, so there are mechanisms in place for your queries.

He convinced us of the vast difference between private and public hospitals in India. After having read Bryan's e-mails describing his experiences in the public hospital (including roaches and no one speaking English), it was quite a stretch for us to imagine something so completely different and with such high standards.

I went straight to the Internet and scoured the Apollo Web site. I read about people from England and other countries who had traveled to New Delhi to have the surgery they would have waited years to have at home. It didn't take much time to figure out that the surgery Howard needed could be done at a fraction of the cost of the same operation performed in the States. I read patients' testimonials about how the hospital had treated them like guests and had taken care of everything from travel to recovery after surgery. I sent an e-mail asking for more information.

We were intrigued with the idea, although we knew very little about India aside from the stereotypes: poverty, cobras, the land of explorers who'd traveled there for spices and silk. Howard had traveled extensively in Europe and South America, and he'd even lived in Antarctica for almost a year. I'd spent months at a time in western Europe and Greece. But India?

Once we opened the "alternatives to U.S. health care" box, it began to fill. Friends from Argentina called to tell us of the expert medical care available there. We asked for more information.

We heard of a doctor in Texas who'd trained at both the Cleveland Clinic and the Mayo Clinic, and has one of the lowest mortality rates in Texas. He had worked out some straight-cash deals with a heart hospital in Texas to attract wealthy patients from Mexico and South America away from Houston. We heard he charged $25 to $35,000 for a valve replacement, including pre-op and hospital costs. I checked out his Web site.

Howard's valve replacement surgery was listed at the lump sum cost of $40,000. I called the office and spoke with a delightful woman who explained everything—the price included all tests, surgery, the hospitalization, and recovery costs. The cardiac surgeon there would be happy to help Howard. The secretary wanted to know how soon we could come. It was simple. Just a domestic plane ticket to Texas and $40,000. We could even use our frequent flyer miles for the plane tickets. The surgeon spoke English. I could stay in a motel chain across the street from the hospital. No big deal.

Then Howard looked at the Web site. The surgeon did more than 650 heart cases each year. "How can any one person do that many operations?" Howard asked. "Sounds like I'd be part of an assembly line." I pictured the canneries many of my friends used to work for in California—tossing rotten tomatoes off the conveyor belt into barrels to make sauce, and allowing the intact ones to ride on by. How far would Howard's heart get to ride?

For some reason, we were both drawn to the option of flying to India, but all of our information had come through Web sites. Then I called a colleague from a biotech company where I used to work. She was Indian, but I didn't know where she was from. She mentioned an article she'd read recently in the *Times of India* about patients coming from all over the world to hospitals in India.

A heart surgeon at Apollo Hospital responded to my e-mail query, suggesting we send the results of Howard's TEE and catheterization tests to him, after Dr. Engel did the procedures in Durham. The soonest Dr. Engel could schedule these tests was still a few weeks away, so we couldn't make any decision about Apollo. But at least we'd had some personal correspondence. We felt one step closer.

My son Bryan's roommate at Stanford was from Hyderabad, a state in southern India, and he was incredibly helpful. He contacted his own travel agent, and offered to carry our visa applications in person to the San Francisco office of the Indian Consulate. His family in India wrote to offer their home to us if we came to their city for the surgery.

Howard got an e-mail from a friend who is a doctor. He said that a robot had been invented to do mitral valve surgery, and the only doctor using it was at East Carolina University in North Carolina, only a two-hour car ride from home. We e-mailed that doctor, who said he would gladly operate on Howard for $70,000. The cost was rising, but it was right here in our own state! We could drive there.

Robot ... robot ... my mind was so jumbled with information ... but I finally cleared a path to my mental connection to "robot." My younger brother, a Ph.D. in mechanical engineering, had helped design the robotic hand featured in the 1980s movie *Short Circuit* while working on his master's degree at the University of Utah. Later, he'd worked on robotic instruments intended to take out the human "tremor" factor during delicate cornea surgery. That was all I could remember. I e-mailed my brother to find out what he knew about the ECU surgeon who used a robot to perform heart surgery.

"Oh, I know Mike," my brother said. "Our company helped design the robot. Every invention needs someone to use it. Engineers can't do heart surgery, so Mike's the surgeon. But it's still in the experimental stage."

"For $70,000 this guy is offering to experiment on Howard's heart?" I asked.

"Well, he's done a lot of them, but there's just not quite enough data." I had always considered my brother's reluctance to voice his opinion as gospel truth an admirable character trait. In this case, it was priceless. When my brother said, "Let's just say, Mike should be paying Howard for the experience," the robot idea was short-circuited right there, on the spot.

We continued to do research and to listen to the opinions of everyone who offered one. Another doctor friend who'd done her residency in China said, "Whatever you do, don't go to India." In fact, the majority of those we spoke to said, "Texas, maybe. But not India! Please."

We got e-mails from doctor friends in major U.S. medical centers who suggested we negotiate with local hospitals—as if they would bid on the opportunity to correct Howard's heart. "They'll never get $200,000 from any insurance company," one from Boston said, "so ask them what they'll do it for." He cited online articles about the real cost of mitral valve surgery, and how hospital costs are figured in the first place.

The Boston doctor summarized the articles for us: "Hospital costs for mitral valve surgery run about $14,000 (not including physician fees, which generally add another 30 to 50 percent). In the first article, "cost" meant "what it cost them"—and then, only directly. Cost was calculated by using operating room, intensive care unit, and ward expenses, not hospital charges.

Not only did this not include physician fees, it didn't include the hospital's profit, i.e., whatever they have to add to cover underpayment by the insurance companies, and tons of other stuff.

The second article showed an average across time and geography. What this average explained was what it would cost to have it done in the U.S. A better way to find that out is just to ask Duke or the University of North Carolina or whomever you want to do the procedure," our friend suggested. "It doesn't matter if the U.S. average is $40,000, if Duke wants to charge $75,000 or whatever. Hospital charges run from $30 to $45,000 (not including physician fees, which, again, generally add another 30 to 50 percent). Insurers pay about a third of this amount at best."

Having already applied that rationale and failed, we still contacted other nearby hospitals. Howard made an appointment with a social worker at the University of North Carolina's Memorial Hospital. They wanted to see his tax returns, financial statements, pay stubs; all were needed to head down the path of Howard qualifying for Medicaid.

While all this was unfolding, Howard turned to his work. I cancelled appointments with my clients, and prepared my students for the possibility of my having to cancel my fall painting and poetry classes. I turned to the information that was pouring in; I embraced it, as if by mulling it over long enough, the solution would appear written upon my wall.

Bryan sent an e-mail to Dr. Srivastava, his professor, who divided his time between Stanford and India and who had firsthand knowledge of health care in both places. He introduced us, described Howard's predicament, and asked for Dr. Srivastava's advice. "What would you decide if it were your own family?" Bryan asked him.

The answer came almost as clearly as I had imagined it would if I just polished our crystal ball of alternatives long enough. Apollo was a fine choice, but he would like to suggest Escorts Heart Institute and Research Center, also in New Delhi.

"To answer your question," Dr. Srivastava wrote to Bryan from India, "if I had a family member in the U.S. who was in a similar position, I would not hesitate to recommend them to come to India for treatment. Indeed, my family and I have a fair share of our health care and treatment here in India. Dr. Naresh Trehan, the founder of Escorts, is of the highest caliber, trained in New York City."

I felt like the raffle box just clicked shut. Time's up. And I was holding the winning ticket. Escorts. This felt like a solution. It felt right. It felt like one of those irrational, unexplainable nods of agreement I sometimes feel in my gut. Still, I googled every way I could think of to investigate Escorts and Dr. Naresh Trehan. I read articles about him and by him. And I finally let go of researching him after reading his name along with Deepak Chopra's in the same sentence, which described luminaries of the twentieth century.

But we couldn't just get on a plane, arrive at this hospital, and sit outside Dr. Trehan's office demanding surgery. Using the address I found on their Web site, I e-mailed them. No response. I tried sending an e-mail request to their "Ask a Cardiologist" page on their Web site. Days passed and we talked again to the Texas doctor.

We downloaded Health Care Power of Attorney forms and filled them out, just to say we did, with no real certainty that anything we signed here would help us in another state or foreign country.

I wrote a letter to Dr. Engel describing our deliberations. I said, "It's between Texas and India. But we want you on board when we come back. We want your blessing."

Howard had another appointment with Dr. Engel. We talked with her nurse about our options. She warned us about the need to learn the customs of other countries. She told us about her daughter who'd had an unexpected hospital experience while traveling in a South American country;

she'd learned that it was customary for the patient's family to provide meals for the entire surgical team.

Then Dr. Engel walked in. "So," she said. "Texas sounds good ..." We waited. "... but I'd go to India."

I think Howard and I began jumping up and down, at least, mentally. It was the choice we wanted to make, but were afraid to without some confirmation and without Dr. Engel's endorsement.

"I've talked with my colleagues," she said. "What you've learned about the facilities in Delhi apparently is right. They are mostly U.S.-trained doctors who have returned to India."

Now it was just a matter of a personal invitation from Escorts Heart Institute. We waited. Days passed. I was impatient. Howard was avoiding the decision. Finally, he said, "Let's just go to Texas and get it over with." The rollercoaster ride of looking for the right answer.

I called the Texas doctor's office. We scheduled the surgery for the following week. The doctor would do the TEE and catheterization himself, and would make his own decision about the kind of surgery Howard needed, thank you very much. And Ooops—the price had gone up to $45,000 instead of the $40,000 posted on the Web site. Howard was too tired to quibble. "I'll be able to pay it off in time."

"But you need it in cash up front," I reminded him. I pictured us walking into the hospital with $45,000 in a plastic baggie.

"Howard," I said, "What if you pay that much, then he does the tests, and he doesn't agree that your mitral valve needs to be repaired or replaced?" I got back on the phone and asked the secretary that question. She agreed we could pay $6,000 until the TEE and catheterization results were in. Then, we could pay the balance, before the surgery.

Deal.

Neither of us was enthusiastic about the decision, but at least it was made. We would go to Texas.

That was when Jackie, my friend and the designer of my Web site, created the site that we named "Howard's Heart" (www.howardsheart.com). I wrote the story. We would use the site to communicate with all of our family and friends for the week or two that we would be in Texas. Sort of like Xeroxed Christmas letters you stuff in with each card. I planned to write one e-mail to Jackie, she would post it on the Web site, and everyone could stay informed.

Predictably, instead of sleeping, I wrestled with the unsettled feeling about submitting Howard's mind and body to something that didn't feel perfect. Dr. Srivastava had given me Dr. Trehan's e-mail address. So, I e-mailed Dr. Trehan myself, and told him we wanted to come to India. No response. Nothing. I wanted to shake the computer to force an e-mail to pop up from Escorts. Nothing.

Then, one night, I was standing in the kitchen when the phone rang. It was 1:00 A.M. Naturally, I thought one of my children had been hurt, or that something had happened to Mom or Dad.

"Maggi? This is Dr. Trehan at Escorts."

Those few words were like a break in the dark sky when you see that first streak of blue after days of hard rain. For still unarticulated reasons, both Howard and I had hoped for India. Dr. Trehan was casual but confident. His assistant would meet us at the airport—we just needed to call him when we knew our flight number. They would do all the tests themselves. Everything would be included.

"And Dr. Trehan," I began, suddenly timid, "I must ask you about the cost. I know you won't know exactly until you do the surgery, but how much money should we bring?"

"You're right. It is difficult to say exactly. It depends on what we find. But I would say that everything will cost no more than eight or nine...," he paused, "let's say to be safe, ten thousand U.S. dollars."

"For everything?" I asked. Of course, we were still sure we would have two or three weeks after the surgery when we planned to go to the beach at Goa or to some mountain retreat to recover. And we knew we would have to pay for that separately, but I repeated, "Everything at Escorts?"

"Absolutely everything," he said.

We sent a rush order to Washington, D.C., for visas to travel to India. I deliberated over writing in "heart surgery" as the trip's purpose, hoping it didn't sound as though we were getting a group together to all have heart surgery at the same time. When the form asked when we would return, I said a little prayer ... to someone ... anyone who might hear it.

Sally, our travel agent friend in Minneapolis, got on the plane tickets immediately. We had to pull out a return date from our thinnest imaginings but finally agreed on a one-month stay, knowing we could change the return if necessary. September 23 through October 24, 2004—who would have thought we would be traveling to India? The cost of each ticket began at $1,700 and went down to $1,300 over the course of a few e-mails.

I don't know what kind of magic Sally was performing, but after experiencing the scope of the foresight she exercised to anticipate needs we didn't even know we might have, I realized her name wasn't Sally Hart simply by coincidence. It is unsettling how words and names seem to jump out at you in different costumes when your focus hones in on something like repairing a heart.

Bryan educated me about the local health centers in the U.S. that are designated as Travel Centers, special facilities that keep up-to-date recommendations from the Centers for Disease Control (CDC) for inoculations and vaccines considered necessary for travel to any foreign country. Online and long distance, Bryan helped identify the Travel Center in Durham I should go to.

Before Howard and I left, I ran around paying medical technicians to shoot vaccines into my arm for diseases I'd only read about in *National Geographic*. Polio I associate with grade school when we lined up to eat sugar cubes, then ducked under our desks to practice what to do when bombs dropped. Tetanus made me think of the time my brother stepped on a rusty nail. And all I remember about malaria was learning to spell tsetse fly for the seventh-grade science test.

I got a shot against hepatitis A at the Durham County Health Department, but had to visit a walk-in Travel Center for the other shots. They were careful to inform me that my Blue Cross Blue Shield health insurance policy would not cover these expenses since they were preventative measures. Because of the short time we had left before leaving, I was too late to get adequate resistance/immunity to some diseases. But I got what I could. I understood very little.

A friend offered to help pay for the drugs. Blue Cross wouldn't. I had to decide between the oral typhoid vaccine that I should have begun taking weeks ago and would have to be refrigerated on the plane, and a shot. I chose the shot. Howard's health was our main concern—I was just trying to take precautions against my getting some disease that would render me helpless to help him.

Just to keep us really preoccupied during this week of waiting for visas, plane tickets, and appointments for the necessary inoculations, my parents were also scheduled to close on the sale of their country home only fifteen minutes away. They were moving to a retirement home. My sister flew up from Florida to help. Emotions ran high and tested our coping skills because we were all facing dramatic life changes—moving, retirement, major surgery, travel to a third-world country—probably all on the list of the top ten stressors.

My parents, both experiencing physical mobility problems, emptied their sunny 2,000 square foot home on two acres with a swimming pool and extensive gardens. After yard sales, classified ads, and an auctioneer to sell off much of their furniture and personal belongings, they filled a climate-controlled storage unit, my attic, and their new two-bedroom apartment with all they thought they'd need for the rest of their lives.

My mother gave up her pots and pans, trading in her life-time duty of cooking for a rigid schedule of three meals a day served in the retirement home's dining room. My father sold his riding lawn mower and many of his tools that I remembered from when I was in grade school. He would no longer have a yard, garage, or workbench. And in one morning, the movers arrived, a housecleaner cleaned their house, and we all crammed into their new place in time for lunch at 12:30 P.M.

That afternoon, I curled up on their love seat in their new apartment, shivering and pale from the side effects of one or more of my travel shots. My mother covered me with an afghan. This would be the place I would picture whenever I thought of going home to Mom and Dad.

A few days later, our visas came. I was glad I had disclosed the real reason for our trip. As our local newspaper would say in their "Roses and Raspberries" column, "Roses to the bureaucrats who must have pushed their visa applications through." Howard's massage therapist, who had gotten him back to work after back surgery, worked us both over thoroughly in preparation for our long flight to India. At the end of Howard's session, he said, "It's on me." At the end of my massage, when I opened my checkbook, he said, "Take care of each other. This is the least I can do."

One night when I could have been asleep, I wrote a poem for Howard. He asked me to see if Jackie could post it on the Web site.

Open Hearted
(for Howard, September 13, 2004)

Poets avoid cliché topics
like butterflies, love, hearts,
but if I wrote to your valve,
readers might think this
an auto parts poem.
The doctor speaks of your heart
as a parachute, your breath
filling it to a high white cloud,
falling on exhale like silk around ankles.
Your anchor strings have snapped
and blood fills your lungs
where air is meant to be clear
as sky before the jump.
You need a seamstress, she says,
and I imagine delicate tatting
and spinning of broken threads,
but here at home, at a price
beyond anyone's cache,

beyond the choice between your heart
or college tuition for your son.
So we must fly days long into tomorrow
to the land of spices and silk.
We will fly
we fly,
so your heart will open
and you may fly.

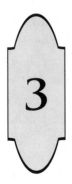

3

SUCCESS ... OR
SO IT SEEMS

Sunday, September 26, 2004

We did fly. And now, I find myself in this land of roadside
food stands and puddles of urine, making my way back to
Howard's hospital room in New Delhi, a Kit Kat bar in my
pocket. A bus pulls up in front of me. People hang off the
sides the way they hang off the cable cars in San Francisco
in the old Rice-A-Roni commercials. Horns are honking in
crossfire. I smell Indian food cooking at a small stand on
wheels. I close my eyes the way I do when I am savoring a
particularly flavorful bite, knowing that, according to Bryan
and every guidebook he ever read, we are not to eat this
food.

Beside the food cart, a little boy dunks huge metal platters into garbage cans full of water to rinse food off the dishes people have eaten from. They look like individual pizza pans, and he stacks them again on the ledge of his father's booth. People walk by, stop and grab a metal plate, and hold it out for food the vendor serves. I walk around the bus and look up.

There it is way up high, the white sign with the big red heart, Escorts Heart Institute and Research Center. I cross the street and walk until I see the guard at the tall iron gate. He watches me as I approach him, tips his hand to his hat. I stuff the Kit Kat bar into my fanny pack, and carry only the markers and rolled-up paper in my hands. I hope they won't search me at the elevator doors. I make it to the fourth floor, nodding hello to everyone I pass. I keep walking until I reach our room, where I notice for the first time that Howard's door is the only one that says "Do Not Disturb." Since we know absolutely no one in India, I wonder who is being protected from whom.

Sunday night in New Delhi. We name this evening Surgery Eve. Howard is instructed to shower with some red soap. Twice. I borrow scissors from the sisters' station, and trim the ends of his hair. Then he trims mine. We never had time for those details before leaving town. I'm sure neither of us has trimmed our toenails in weeks.

A social worker comes for a briefing about postsurgical care. We will stay in the hospital five to seven days, then somewhere in the nearby area. The rules are:

1. Do not drive or work for three months.

2. Ride only in the backseat.

3. Lift up on knees with hands to stand up.

4. Roll over to get up and out of bed—no strain on the heart.

After an incredible feast on bedside trays, lunch today acts as a strong sedative for both of us. We both nap hard. Is this the calm before the storm?

The man in white comes again, and motions for Howard to follow him. He returns about twenty minutes later in his karate uniform. "I'm a plucked chicken," Howard says. But I can see his ponytail still intact. "They got everything but the hair on my head."

"Everything?"

Howard nods that goofy grin of his where he shifts his lips to one side. "From the tip of me nose to the hair on me toes." He stands in the middle of the room, unties the string on his wraparound top, and drops his pants to the floor. "Even the hair on me arse!" I've seen newborn babies that have the faces of old men, but never have I seen a grown man in a baby's body. With his dark hair gone, he is pale, shiny, and downright skinny! Skin I have never seen bare looks soft and tender. "I reckon they fancy me a plucked chicken, I do."

I can't imagine the philosophy behind shaving toes for heart surgery, but I want to hear all about how it was done. Howard explains the entire procedure to me.

"This guy is an expert. Used a five-inch blade with a five-inch handle—stainless steel—to make long sweeps and swipes. The hair fell off; he moved it away with one hand, and checked for skin tags with one eye. This guy is extremely good."

Howard is shaved cleaner than he's been since birth. We are both impressed with the barber's artistry.

"I was lying on a table, but he is so short, he stood on a stool. He held each nipple to shave around. Held my dick and balls—shaved me clean as a pig's whistle." I hear pride in Howard's voice, or perhaps it is sheer respect. "I tipped him," he says. "Fifty rupees."

"Is that the going rate for plucking a chicken?" I ask.

The Barber

On the eve of surgery, you bathe
twice with a bucket of red soap.
A slim Hindu summons you
to the corner of the ward, to step
behind his windowless door.
In white uniform with black stripes,
thick white sox and gray sandals,
he will prepare you for morning.

He sets his toolbox on the floor, opens
the mirrored lid, sets free clouds of orange
blossom to fill the tiny room. When you close
your eyes, you see silhouettes of your chin
multiplied against pumpkin-colored walls.

You motion a warning, a plea for his steady hand
to navigate your hiccups. He nods. Sir,
no problem, Sir. The dark man opens his blade,
holds it in an L while he steadies your head
with his left hand—thumb pressing up at your temple,
two fingers spread your skin taut. Eyes still closed,
you follow breaths in and out to catch up
to the hiccups, while he shaves you dry from ears

to tops of toes. He must not weigh 100 pounds,
but holds wisdom of skin, of obstacles and curves.

Finally he grips a cone of antiseptic ice, paints
your skin until you glisten like a buttered turkey.
He blots the spots of blood with tissue, then rubs
his hands with Dettol, pats your face, chest, groin,
smoothes you down with a dry towel. Ceremoniously
he folds the towel like a flag, and says, *No pain.*

You see it is a question. You tip him 50 rupees
and the answer. *No pain,* you say, seeing his feet
in the mirror, covered in your hair. In the morning,
How many rupees will you hide under your cap?

By the time dinner arrives, Howard and I awake from
our second nap. Howard discovers two Kit Kat bars under a
napkin on his tray. His plea has reached someone downstairs.
I realize my treat was not so special after all, smuggling or
not. Maybe whoever makes Kit Kats has a monopoly in the
Indian market, and it's the only candy bar available.

Tonight, Howard writes a letter to his son, Alan, which
I am to hand-deliver should anything go wrong tomorrow. I
think back to the tagline of "if there are no complications."
We sit on his bed and do a simple meditation. We draw
mandalas with the markers I bought—circular symbols of
what we pray for. Howard's is of a tree with a sleeping man
beneath the branches—napping, of course. Peaceful. Mine is
of Dr. Trehan's eyes and hands, hovering over an orange sun
for the purest judgment.

Sister Josi brings him two sedatives. "Nothing to eat or
drink for Mr. Howard." And she instructs me to watch, in

case he gets up to pee. Finally about 1:15 A.M., Howard falls asleep.

Monday, September 27, 2004

About 6:00 A.M. Howard gets up to pee. This is the day. Coffee comes, then breakfast for both of us. It is a mistake. We agree that Howard is not to eat. I ask the sisters, but they say Howard's surgery is not until tomorrow. A team of cardiologists comes to examine Howard and tells us the surgery will be this afternoon. They are waiting for one more test. The more people we ask, the more certain we are that no one really knows. Finally, someone calls Dr. Trehan. The report is: No surgery today. The tests are not back. Surgery will be first thing in the morning.

Communication at its best. The kind of disappointment you feel when you hear the doctors will not cut open your heart today is difficult to describe. Even more of a challenge is how to spend another twenty-four hours "resting" when you have nothing to rest from.

We walk the halls, check e-mail, and Howard writes his own e-mails to Alan and his closest friend, Rob. I think feeling like a plucked chicken is the highlight of his trip so far. Though neither Howard nor I watch television at home, we try it here. No English subtitles on the Indian sitcoms or movies, so the only thing worth checking is CNN. We work more crossword puzzles, read our books. Howard finishes *Holy Cow*, by Sarah Macdonald, the story about a journalist's wife surviving in Delhi while her husband travels for a story.

Today is Bryan's birthday—my older son turns twenty-three today (or yesterday or tomorrow, depending on how good I am at figuring the time change), and here I am in India. Both of my sisters in Florida survived another hurricane—Hurricane Jeanne. Life as usual. And life as usual can seem awfully long when you know that life will change in the morning. At least Howard can eat, and we drag out each meal as if it were the "Last Supper."

Tuesday, September 28, 2004

The sisters come in early and again ask Howard to bathe twice with the special red shampoo, then put on a clean outfit. Only one food tray comes for me; nothing for Howard. Finally, this day feels different from the others. I comb Howard's hair and braid it, fastening the braid with two elastic bands for extra security.

I tell Howard about the surgeon I used to work for who wrote silly things on the penises of patients he knew well while they were anesthetized. When they awoke from surgery, they were always surprised at what word sprang to life upon first erection.

"Let's surprise these Indian doctors," Howard says.

"How 'bout just thank you?" I suggest.

I have already asked someone to write down the correct spelling in my little notebook. We write "dhanyawaad," the Hindi word for "thank you," across Howard's chest on the right side for the surgical team. I use the purple marker.

The sisters return accompanied by an attendant with a gurney. One sister puts a surgical cap on Howard's head, tucking in his braid. While Howard listens to the CD of Joni Mitchell's "Both Sides Now," Sister Deepti inserts the access for an IV.

I play the game, "Who loves Howard?"

He says, "You love me, Alan does, Will and Molly do, Mom and Dad, Donna, Sarina, and especially Susan, Vince, Andrew and Neva, Rob and Laura...."

As we have discussed previously, Howard asks me to change the CD to the soundtrack from *O Brother, Where Art Thou?* for the surgery. Sister Reena and Sister Deepti and I follow Howard on his gurney down the hall, into the elevator. He waves to all the sisters at the station when we pass by.

My previous marriage to a surgeon has instilled in me the practice of making sure patients are seen by doctors as people with faces, instead of as just another gallbladder, or the mastectomy in room 235. Outside the Operating Theater, I introduce myself and shake hands with the anesthesiologists and surgeons, all in blue scrubs, who make up Howard's team. (Of course, this will include Dr. Trehan, though he is not among this group yet.) I look straight into the eyes of the one I suspect is the head anesthesiologist and say, "If you put him to sleep, you wake him up. Okay?"

"Of course. Do not worry. He will do fine." He smiles. I don't.

And if Howard doesn't wake up, I want this guy to know what I look like and where to find me.

"I will be in Howard's room on the fourth floor," I say. "I'm not leaving without him."

Howard sings along with his tape at the top of his lungs—a song about living and dying—and we hear every word because Howard doesn't stutter when he sings. I lean down and press my cheek to Howard's, then interrupt his singing to kiss him. "You might have to leave your banjo with me," I say. "See you in the morning. I love you."

One doctor tries to take away the Discman and earphones, but I insist Howard keep them. "Okay, but only until he is asleep," he concedes. I nod.

One of the anesthesiologists holds up Howard's X-ray and says to me, "He has a very strong heart."

"And a very strong will," I add, as they wheel him into the Operating Theater.

"They go together," he says. And I am, for the first time, thankful for Howard's stubbornness. The double doors close behind the last of the men in blues.

Reena and Sister Deepti and I are left standing in the lobby. Such a long road to get here; and there is no turning back. I don't try to dry the tears spilling down my face. It is only a few minutes before a doctor pushes through the doors again and hands me Howard's Discman.

Tuesday Afternoon

It is 3:15 in the afternoon, and the busy street parade I watch from our fourth-floor window is like a river—an ever-changing flow of cows, rickshaws, building materials, and colorful saris, while at the same time remaining a constant recognizable entity. If I let my eyes glaze over, the scene I return to when I focus again is the same, as if I'd accidentally hit pause in a DVD.

I count the hours again. More than six since those wide double doors to the operating theater closed behind Howard's gurney and he gazed back at me sideways standing there in the foyer. They said four to six hours. I want to hear some word from the doctors. Even if they aren't finished, I know someone can relay a progress report to me. Sometimes patients are in Recovery for a long time before the doctors remember to go and report to the family. The risk of being annoying trumps my patience. I walk down to the sisters' station. I make a pretend phone gesture with hand to ear, to ask Sister Deepti to call Recovery for me.

She looks at me and says, "Everything is fine." But I point to an imaginary watch on my wrist and hold up six fingers. I know my eyes can't hide my worry. Sister Deepti phones, the only words I recognize imbedded in her conversation are "Mr. Howard." Suddenly she sets the phone down with one hand, motions to another sister in white to take me downstairs.

My heart seems audible in the elevator, but I follow Sister Anjuli down long hallways into a small room lined with cubbies similar to the ones my children used at pre-school. She hands me a pair of gray rubber sandals. I slip off my shoes and put my feet into the sandals with only a fleeting thought about how many people have worn these before me. I follow Anjuli through more doors, down more hallways, until we come to a swinging glass door. She motions to a short bin of paper masks. I place one over my mouth and tie it behind my head. My hands are shaking. When I look up, I see the ends of several beds in a row, and lots of nurses and doctors scattered around this open room I will come to know as "Recovery." I step inside as if it were an underground chapel I have finally discovered.

I feel like an intruder, a voyeur, but force myself to look at the faces of the patients, trying to locate Howard. I see him: middle bed on the right. A tube that reminds me of a dryer vent hangs out of the right side of his mouth. His neck is at least a size 20 (five sizes up from this morning when I gathered his hair to braid it). His eyes are shut tight, glistening with thick grease. My eyes sting. The room blurs. I cannot see above the mask now. I imagine Howard breaking out into some off-key rendition of "Drown in My Own Tears." But this is the first and last time I forget to bring tissues in a pocket or tucked into my bra. I am thankful for long loose sleeves.

Tubes protrude straight out from the left side of Howard's neck and wrap around his head. I think of Medusa's snakes, and then try to shake the macabre image. His hair is no longer neatly braided or even tucked up inside the blue shower cap, but tousled around his face, stuck to his skin in clumps. I keep staring at his neck. The tubes, too many to count, protrude as if they'd grown there naturally. I am reminded of Atul Gawande's stories in *The New Yorker* about learning to perform these techniques as a young surgical resident. I wonder how many pokes it takes before the average doctor gets used to directly piercing or slicing a patient's flesh.

I don't want to take my eyes off Howard, but finally I look at the doctor who stands at the foot of Howard's bed with a clipboard in hand. In a cloud of broken English and Hindi, and with me repeating every word to make sure I have all the information right, I learn (or think I learn) that the procedure went as planned. They were able to repair the mitral valve; they did not have to replace it.

What I hear is that they used a standard "ring" procedure called "the Hopper method," going intercostally through the ribs instead of having to perform a sternotomy, which would have cut through the sternum. (I still have visions of a doctor with goggles on, standing over Howard with a tool belt draped around his hips, revving a chainsaw before dropping it down in the center of his chest in one smooth cut.)

I can feel my own chest heave with the breath I must have been holding for the last six hours. I replay Dr. Engel's description of the options back home. Howard will heal more quickly this way. He will be in less pain than if he'd had his sternum sliced in half. Had we stayed in North Carolina and gone this route, Howard would be at Duke University Medical Center under the care and knife of the surgeon most expert in this less-invasive technique. We never got to meet him.

I quickly remember my job: to gather and record information that Howard cannot possibly ask for now. The ventilator is set for 12 (Is that good? What is normal?), and it is breathing for him so he can rest. I ask about the bypass machine, blood lost, blood required. He had been on the heart-lung bypass machine for only 118 minutes and used only one pint of blood during surgery. Doctors and nurses qualify this point more than once over the next few days, reminding me that Howard might require additional blood during recovery. (Of course, I know he won't. If he didn't bleed during surgery, he certainly won't start bleeding now. After all, he will be up and walking tomorrow, and we will be out of here in just a couple more days.) Again, I hear Dr. Engel's instruction at the end of our last visit. "Get him up, Maggi. No matter what they say over there, get him up walking as soon as you can after surgery. No matter what."

I continue my data collection: His blood pressure is slightly elevated (132/80), which they tell me is normal right after surgery. I ask about each crimson number on the monitor above the head of his bed until I learn enough to recognize the changes that will alter this story all too soon. For now, Howard's pulmonary function is good, no arrhythmia (his heart is beating regularly on its own—the monitor says 107 beats per minute instead of his usual pulse of 70). Yes, Howard is on antibiotics. The next visiting time is 6:00 P.M.

I stand motionless as the doctor moves on to the next patient. The sister at the end of Howard's bed is stationed at a music stand, charting numbers by hand on pages and pages of huge yellow graph paper. How can there be this much to write down already? Especially about a patient for whom everything went well, for someone who will be up and walking down the hall tomorrow? I suddenly remember Sister Anjuli who escorted me down here. I look back at the glass door, and there she stands, as if she hasn't moved one step because no one told her to. She doesn't look impatient at having waited this long.

I follow Sister Anjuli down the same hallways, retracing our path back "home." We pass a receptacle for our used masks, go back through the shoe cubby room and change shoes, pass the guard at the elevator, and arrive back up on the fourth floor.

Sister Deepti faces me as I come around the corner. "Mr. Howard is fine," I say. She smiles, holds her hands together, looks up and says, "Thank god." I haven't even asked her which god she thanks.

A sister follows me to my room and unlocks my door. It has been a long day, but the difficult part is behind us. The decision to repair the valve was made; the surgery is over and was successful. Now, Howard will simply rest and heal. Then we will hop a train to the beaches we read about in the guidebook.

My patient tray table is in front of the window with my four o'clock thermoses of tea and coffee. (The sisters confiscated a second tray table from who-knows-where so that Howard and I could eat sitting side by side on the sofa.) Today, there is a round biscuit on my tray in a waxed paper wrapper. Yes, a special treat. I have so much to celebrate, so much to be grateful for.

The term "watch the clock" takes on a more expansive meaning, as I don't dare close my eyes, for fear I will miss the magic hour of 6:00 P.M.: official visiting hours for patients in Recovery.

I feel the butterflies of adolescent anticipation. Even Cinderella comes to mind. I want to abide by the house rules as much as I can, knowing I can and will defy them if they prevent me from getting information I need or in any way compromise Howard's care. I allow time (about seven minutes) to greet all of the sisters and security guards as I make my way through the hallways, wait for the elevator, change my shoes, tie on a face mask, and enter Recovery at exactly six o'clock. This time, I travel unassisted. This is a legitimate visit.

I go directly to Howard, bed number two. I try to find one plain section of his head to touch, then speak in his ear loud enough to penetrate his deep sedated sleep. "I love you, Howard. I love you so much. Everything went well, and all you have to do now is rest." I have forgotten how awkward it feels to talk to someone who cannot acknowledge me, let alone respond. Suddenly, I run out of things to say. "I love you, Howard. Everything's going to be...." His eyes flutter so slightly I wonder if it is an involuntary response. Then he squeezes my hand! He hears me! I feel as though I am in some sappy movie watching for signs of life. Typically, Howard smiles so much and so often, that it strikes me as especially peculiar to feel his response, to know he is glad I am next to him, and to see no facial expression at all.

But the hand squeeze is all it takes for me to continue to speak to him, to stroke his forehead, to squeeze his hand. I have a hundred questions to ask him, and another hundred things to tell him—about the men who came to pee against the wall today, about the carpenters on bicycles carrying bricks in their pockets, about the one unit of blood he needed during surgery, about the Hopper technique, about my needing to learn the name of the lime green birds in the trees outside our window, about the cookie on my tray at tea time. "Everything is fine, Howard. I'm right here."

Dimple is his Recovery nurse this afternoon. I use my imaginary watch again, and she tells me she leaves at 8:00 P.M. I speak with Dr. Mishra, the attending physician in the Recovery Room. He explains that Howard's blood pressure and heart rate are good. He is still on the ventilator. "It takes time to wake up," he says. "He must rest. You can come tomorrow at noon."

"Noon?" I feel the house rules rising in my way. I kiss Howard's forehead. "I'll be just upstairs in our room," I say. "Just rest now. Pretend I'm right next to you." I return to our room, to our window.

With nothing but time, I stare. I think, until a shadow of unease enfolds me. I'm accustomed to surgical patients being moved to the Recovery Room after their operation simply to be stabilized—an hour or so, tops. Then they are moved to their room. I realize Dr. Trehan has not come to our room to talk to me about Howard's surgery. But I remind myself of how busy Dr. Trehan must be. And I remind myself that I spoke to Dr. Mishra. Dr. Trehan will probably come to see both of us tomorrow when Howard is transferred up to our room. For now, I must try to get sleepy.

I work on a crossword puzzle that Howard and I left unfinished. A friend of a friend of Howard's phones me from Jodhpur to check on Howard's condition. Our communication is difficult but meaningful. He promises to call every day.

Mr. Sanjiv, my personal liaison it seems, visits me, asks about Mr. Howard. When I explain that the surgery went well and that Howard is resting, Sanjiv takes my hands in his and nods in assurance. "Of course," he says, then "Thank god." He releases my hands and says, "And now, what will you eat, Indian veg?"

He suspects I will stick with the usual, but I ask, "What else is there?" I have eaten Indian veg three meals a day for the last five days.

"Anything you want," he says. "You want Continental? Chinese?"

This is the first I've heard of Chinese. "Chinese? They have Chinese here?"

He nods. "Anything you want. You want Chinese? You have Chinese. Tonight."

It seems almost sacrilegious to eat Chinese in this Indian hospital. But I feel like eating something new, to celebrate. "Yes, Chinese veg, please," I say. "Thank you."

Sanjiv has the slightest look of disappointment on his face, but I convince myself he doesn't give a rat's ass what I eat. He is just doing his job. Probably can't wait to get out of here and go home. "See you tomorrow," he says. "Good night."

"Good night." I think of him as he closes my door behind him. So mysteriously quiet, always appearing out of nowhere, at my doorway, at the elevator the time I tried to visit the lobby downstairs without a pass. I wonder if someone kisses him good-bye at the door when he leaves in the morning; if someone waits for him at this hour.

Surely he has a wife with dark eyes, waiting in a flowing silk sari, her black hair so shiny it lights up the dark. The dining table is probably covered with a cloth of bright color, set with an assortment of small silver pans with lids—all separate dishes of rice, dal, nan, paneer this, and masala that, delicately simmered so the scents in the house swirl with spices that seem at once separate and perfectly blended.

I try to imagine Sanjiv without his starched shirt and tie, wonder if he wears shorts and a T-shirt at home. This thought is so out of character it makes me smile, as if I were fantasizing about him with his clothes off. I don't, of course, and pull myself back to the image of Howard's eyes weighted down with Vaseline, his swollen face and neck, his puffy, taut hands. I suddenly don't care about Chinese. I want to sit beside Howard's bed. I want to be there when his eyes are strong enough to shed that layer of grease.

The door opens again, and it is Medha, the woman from the Information Desk, asking if I need anything. Anything at all. Until now, my answer has been, "No, we are fine." I have been unable to imagine anything I need that they don't bring me without my asking. But tonight I want to talk to my mom and dad. "Yes, please. I would like to call the U.S."

Medha bobs her head from side to side, like a gentle shaking of water from the ears, a gesture I have come to know as a sign of agreement, or "okay," "sure," or "fine" instead of "no." "One moment, please." She walks over to my phone, her high heels clicking, and dials. In very quick Hindi, I recognize only two phrases: U.S. and coffee shop. She puts down the receiver and then dials again. Several conversations later, she turns to me. "So," she says, with her hands pressed together. "In morning you buy card at the coffee shop. Then you phone U.S." I'm disappointed by the skewed sense of urgency here. Tomorrow. Today. There seems to be no difference here. I thank her and she leaves, closing the door gently behind her, as if I am engaged in some top secret activity and need my privacy.

My activity is waiting. I am waiting—as publicly and actively as I have ever waited in my life—except perhaps for that blustery September afternoon twenty-three years ago when I was in labor, and my then-husband walked me around the block, stopping to pant in unison with me every third driveway.

Here, I try to understand, and then wait, and hope I did indeed understand what the doctor said correctly; I try to think of questions I forgot to ask. It still doesn't occur to me that if we were back home in North Carolina, I would return to the waiting room to relay all the information I learned in the Recovery Room to my parents, our friends, and Howard's son, Alan. The contrast should be readily apparent since I was one of the 300 friends and relatives to play the waiting game en masse by dominating the lobby of Durham Regional Hospital during my friend's mother's thirty-eight-day recovery.

In retrospect, that extended and frightening time was only tolerable, if it ever was that, by the rotating of night duty, the hundreds of visits from people who love the family, by the food brought in, the games and newspapers and the all-too-infrequent distractions for some of those family members who occasionally returned to their regular jobs. Had I even compared that support group to this solo waiting, I would have panicked. Fortunately, as we often do, I do what is required of me now, and will process it later. What is required of me now is to imagine Howard walking down the hall in his white hospital pajamas, laughing, his long thin braid dividing his back.

ENTERING THE
INNER SANCTUM

Wednesday, September 29, 2004

Wednesday, 7:30 A.M., I wake on my own, shower, and call Recovery. The phone is passed, I imagine, to the sister at Howard's feet, someone other than Dimple, someone I haven't met yet. "He is okay now" is her report. Even in broken English, the word "now" blinks in bright neon.

"What do you mean *now*?" I ask. "How was his night?" I can hear my voice rising.

There is more passing of the phone, and finally a doctor's voice. "We did another echocardiogram, and there was ..."

then the words "resistance," "blood," and "atrium." I don't understand. As if to calm me, the doctor says, "Dr. Trehan will reassess at nine o'clock."

Reassess what? I don't know what has happened, and "okay now" is no comfort at all. I put the phone down. What is magic about nine o'clock? I have never been one to wait to understand. I pace, I huddle on my black sofa and stare down at the street. I weigh the cost of storming into the Recovery Room, demanding an explanation; I wonder if I can wait. But nine o'clock does not necessarily mean nine o'clock. This much I have learned. It could mean noon . . . it could be nine o'clock tomorrow.

Somewhere during my mental calculations, the phone rings. "Please. Come to Recovery." I do not ask anyone to lock my room; I simply shout to Sister Deepti as I pass the station, "I go to Recovery." My heart scares me, it's pounding so hard. I make my way unescorted, through a watery world of hallways and elevators.

When I enter Recovery, a group of doctors and sisters are huddled near the door. I try to pass them to go straight to Howard's bed, but a doctor speaks directly to me. "We did an echo this morning." I force myself to focus on what he is saying. "The anterior cusp has thickened and is causing resistance of blood flow to the body. We must go back in and replace the valve." An electric current shoots through me. My eyes instantly tear up. Everyone is looking at me, but their faces blur.

I wait for more explanation, and then I realize what this announcement means. "A second operation?" I ask. The collage of faces seems to be underwater. Their voices blend into an indistinguishable hum.

"Yes."

"Today?"

"Yes, as soon as we can get him into the Operating Theater."

My legs feel weak, but I force myself to attention. "Can he survive another surgery? Will he be under general anesthesia again?"

"Yes. He will be fine."

Someone hands me a clipboard. "Please sign here." I recognize this instruction. They are asking me to sign a consent form for Howard to have a second operation. I look toward his bed and know he is in no condition to make this decision. But I am not his wife. He is not my child. For a split second I wonder how sure I am that Howard would even say yes.

"Does Howard know?" I ask.

"No. He is not fully awake from the first surgery."

I look at the clipboard. A sister holds out a pen. I take it, try to steady the clipboard. I sign on the line, or at least somewhere near it. "I want to see him before you take him," I say, already walking toward his bed.

"It is best if he does not know," the doctor says. "He must remain calm."

Howard is still swollen, his color still pasty. Tubes and IV lines still tangle around his head and chest, the ventilator still pulls his tongue out to the right side like a tired dog's. But today he opens his eyes and looks at me. With his right hand, he points to the line in his neck and winces with his eyes.

I nod. "You have a line in that side of your neck. I'm sure it doesn't feel good. They'll take it out soon, I'm sure." I'm sure of nothing. I lean down to kiss his forehead, to speak directly into his ear. "Everyone loves you so much, Howard." My eyes fill to the brim. It's impossible to stop the tearing. At least my mask covers my nose and mouth. "I'm staying right here with you. I promise. I'm not going anywhere. I love you." What else can I possibly say? Only clichés, probably every one I've ever heard in a sappy movie or, back in the sixties, when I read *Love Story* on a plane after leaving my boyfriend.

Howard looks down at his hand. I watch as he holds up one finger, then another, then another. He looks at me, all business. I want to rip out the ventilator and just hold him. But he wants to know something. Now. He releases his fingers again the same way, one at a time.

I get it. "Are you asking me how many more hours you have to stay here?" I ask him.

He closes his eyes and I detect a slight frown beginning to appear between his eyebrows. "How many days?" I guess.

I get a yes. I decide instantly that this is one exception to the "information is power" rule. I do not tell him about the new plan to replace his valve. I would never forgive myself if telling him made him anxious, if he did not tolerate the new surgery as well as he might, because I told him. "Very soon," I say. "As soon as you are strong enough, you will come back to the room." I know this is not good enough, but I don't know what else to say. I take his right hand in mine. "I love you so much."

He squeezes my hand for a "me too" sign. His eyes are already closed again.

"You rest now, okay? I will be in our room, and I promise I won't leave the hospital." My tears drop over my mask. My nose is running behind it. I back away from his bed.

The sister at the foot of his bed puts her hand on my shoulder. "He will be fine. God will take care of him." God. God has come and gone in my life, but never have I felt so far away from any concept of a god.

Out in the hall, I untie my mask and use it to wipe my nose. It wasn't supposed to be like this. This has to be one of those complications Mr. Damien and Mr. Finance kept qualifying the $100,000 hospital cost with; "... if there are no complications," they kept saying. No wonder it always made me cringe. I want to throw something, but all I have is this soggy mask. I toss it in a trash barrel.

When I get back to the fourth floor, Sister Deepti is at the desk with several other sisters, some in white, some in brown. I'm still crying, my voice unreliable, but I try to speak deliberately to report, "Mr. Howard is having surgery again."

Two of them walk on either side of me, but do not offer the comfort of touch. The mantra that is more irritating than consoling begins.

"God will take care of him."

"Mr. Howard will be fine."

"Do not cry."

"Trust God."

One sister unlocks my door. "Thank you," I manage to say.

I realize Sister Deepti must have sent someone to lock my door when I ran out of here. They take such fine care of me.

When I'm finally alone on the sofa, I let go of all the checks I'd put in place when I was in the Recovery Room to keep myself from falling apart. I cry a deep cleansing cry. The kind that rattles your body so hard, you let someone hold you even though you're soaking both of your shirts with tears and snot. But there is no one here to hold me. I wrap my arms around my knees. I even begin to rock, ever so slightly.

Breakfast comes but I cannot eat. I just sit with my knees pulled up to my chest, a box of tissues beside me. Sisters come in and ask if I need anything. Every encounter ends with "Do not cry," and "Trust God." But all I can do is cry. All I can wonder is where anyone's God is this time.

I tell random people I've seen Dr. Trehan only once. I tell people who I'm sure do not understand me that in the U.S., doctors come to talk to their patients after surgery—here, you're lucky if they call you. I think of how little I know, and that I just had to sign for more surgery. I think of all the people Howard has known longer than me and I can't believe what I've just done. I try to think of who would argue against the need for more surgery. Who could I possibly ask?

Suddenly Naruna knocks and comes in. I start crying all over again, and he hugs me. I tell him about Howard's second surgery and begin my rant about not seeing Dr. Trehan, about doctors not coming to me to explain what happened.

"Come," he says. "Dr. Trehan wants to see you."

I slip on my white sandals and pluck a few more tissues from the box. I grab my notepad and a pen, hook my reading glasses over the neckline of my blouse. In the elevator, I explain, "With all due respect, I understand it might just be different here. But in America, the doctor comes to the family to explain how the surgery went. I haven't seen Dr. Trehan in days." I start to feel a little more daring. "I'm not even sure he was there for the surgery."

Naruna looks at me with his eyes wide. "Of course he was. You want to talk to him? He will talk to you."

Any clarity I had fades and I can't decide whether I'm angry or sad . . . or just scared to death.

Soon we are standing in a waiting room outside Dr. Trehan's office. He has many guards and assistants, many of whom I recognize from Recovery and from my room. There is a full room of people in street clothes. I am the only white person, which somehow seems more noticeable here. I can't tell if these people are prospective patients, family members of patients, or what. All I can tell is they are waiting. People slip out of Dr. Trehan's office. Someone else is escorted inside. It all looks so official. I'm so tired. So confused.

Before it can possibly be my turn, Naruna motions for me to come with him. Inside this huge office, I quickly scan the layout: chairs and a love seat on one wall, Dr. Trehan's desk facing them. Behind his desk is an entire wall of monitors with vitals being charted, maybe ten or twelve. Dr. Trehan is standing behind his desk. He is in blues with a face mask dangling around his neck.

"*Namaste,*" I say, holding my hands pressed together up to my forehead the way my yoga teacher greets the students and says good-bye to us in class.

"So, you are learning some Hindi?" He smiles. "Please sit down."

Naruna shows me to a chair directly in front of Dr. Trehan's desk. Attendants line up behind Dr. Trehan as he takes his seat. Phones ring, they answer them, and an occasional one gets handed to Dr. Trehan; some attendants just talk in low voices and wait for Dr. Trehan to hold up his hand and accept another phone from behind him. This is a well-rehearsed scene, a seamless relay of information filtered through this one man.

Simultaneously, Dr. Trehan draws on a folded piece of paper and talks to me, talks on one cell phone, hands it back to an assistant, continues to talk to me, accepts another phone—and I never feel neglected. He draws a diagram of the ring procedure they used to repair Howard's mitral valve. He sewed in the ring and cut out the broken chordae. I am reminded of Dr. Engel's parachute metaphor, and her explanation that Howard's chords had snapped.

"The repair was successful," he says.

"And you used the Hopper technique?" I ask.

He looks at me, puzzled. "Hopper?"

I point to my side. "The one you learned in Salt Lake City, going in through the ribs instead of the sternum." I feel so ridiculous—me explaining this to him. I must have terribly misunderstood something important.

He relaxes the scrunched up lines in his forehead and smiles. "Ah, you mean Heart Port."

I am embarrassed. I have misunderstood what Dr. K. explained to me. All this time I imagined there was some Dr. Hopper who'd first tried to repair a heart valve without slicing through the sternum.

Dr. Trehan is amused but not condescending. I'm grateful. "Yes, we went in through the ribs," he says, and continues, darkening the line that separates the heart into two halves. "In 6 percent of valve repairs, the septum thickens and obstructs blood flow to the body," he says. "It is called septal anterior motion." (He writes "S.A.M." on the paper.) "When Howard began to wake up this morning, this happened to him."

"So, before surgery, his blood was gushing out ... and now it is obstructed?" I ask.

"Yes," he says. "It is the opposite problem."

I try hard to pay attention to the information. "Don't start crying," I tell myself. "No crying!" I know the blood must travel from the heart to the rest of his body. There can't be a lot of time left for Howard's heart to remain obstructed. I think of how long a person can survive in freezing cold water *without damage*. That's always the qualifier. I try to remember how long an unborn baby can survive with inadequate blood supply or oxygen, without suffering brain damage. I think of how many babies do survive, and what the damage can be.

"In some instances, we can give patients medicine to try to shrink down the septum or cusp, so there is no obstruction and blood flows freely. But since Howard is not from here, and since I do not want to send him home with a problem that might not correct itself, I think it is best to replace the valve." He is calm. He is confident.

I remember my role, and try to align my questions. "Will you go back in through the same site?"

"Yes."

"Will he have another general anesthetic?"

"Yes."

"When will you do the surgery?"

"We will take him in now," Dr. Trehan says. "Hopefully we will be done by two o'clock."

I look at my watch. It is only 9:30 in the morning. I feel like a lifetime has already passed. I gather energy for all I want to tell Dr. Trehan in case it is my last time. "I did not tell Howard about the second surgery," I say. "I didn't want to upset him. But he asked me how long it would be before he got out of Recovery." Dr. Trehan nods.

"I want to be near Howard as soon as I can, after this is over." He nods again. I continue, "I think he will feel less anxious if I'm there. And he wants to hear music as soon as possible, too." I dig for anything else I want to know or need to say. I finally point to the sketch he has made of the valves and ask, "May I keep this please?"

"Of course." He hands me the diagram of Howard's heart.

"Thank you very much for your time," I say. Clutching the paper, I press the palms of my hands together again. "Namaste."

Naruna and I leave and pass all the people still waiting outside Dr. Trehan's office. The sense of guilt I feel for receiving preferential treatment tries to interrupt my new calm, but I shoo it away. I will gladly take whatever edge we have for being the first Americans, no matter how unfair it may be. I need to get Howard well and back home. Naruna walks me back to my room. "Going to see Dr. Trehan is like going to see the Wizard of Oz," I say in the elevator.

It never crosses my mind that Naruna might not know who or where Oz is. Then I suddenly realize all those monitors represent the patients Dr. Trehan watches from his office—maybe those newly out of surgery, maybe all those in Recovery.

A sister unlocks my room. Naruna notices the mandalas taped to our closet door. "Did you draw these?" he asks.

I explain how the night before surgery, Howard and I made the mandalas. "We wrote our intention on the backs, then meditated, thinking about that intention," I say. "Then we drew whatever images came to mind to make that intention come true."

Naruna looks at mine of Dr. Trehan's eyes and hands above a blazing orange sun. "May I take this to Dr. Trehan?" he asks.

I take it down and give it to him. He turns it over to read my intention: That Howard would have no fear, that the healing process would begin now. That Dr. Trehan's eyes would focus, his judgment be clear, and his hands expert.

When Naruna leaves, I repeat to myself over and over what Dr. Trehan explained and I try to write it down so I can tell Howard. I'm filled with dread at having to e-mail everyone back home and tell them what's happened—afraid they will think we made a mistake in coming here, afraid they will assume Dr. Trehan didn't do a good job. But I'm confident that Dr. Trehan was right—that the repair was successful—but that Howard's body did that S.A.M. thing.

I can't remember what it stands for, but want to look it up online. It sounds like an individual's natural response; like being allergic to some substance or having a keloid form at the site of an injury or incision where the wound heals with excessive, bulky scar tissue. I remember the time the plastic surgeons I once worked for argued over the best way to remove a wart on my hand. The chief burned it off, then the junior partner assured me if he cut it out and stitched it up, I'd have an almost invisible single-line scar. I let him do it, but in the end, the scar widened and thickened. The junior partner was off the hook, though. "You didn't tell me you were a keloider," he said.

I decide I will not e-mail anyone until Howard is safely recovering again. What would be the point? I am also acutely aware of the hours that lie ahead of me. Knowing I can't read a novel when I am worried, I get out my Swiss Army Knife and begin to cut words out of newspapers. I will make a collage for Howard. I'm grateful for the tiny scissors that I've rarely used in the thirty years of owning this knife. Snipping headlines like "Brave," "Heart," and "Chocolate," I make a pile of tear-soaked Howard-words that look like confetti or packing material.

I also review Dr. Trehan's words. Surely Howard would not opt for being on medication for months to try to shrink the obstructing septum. He hates medicine, hates to be restricted at all. And he might end up needing to have the valve replaced anyway. I'm convinced Howard would want to get the new valve and get on with his life. If only he survives this back-to-back general anesthesia.

I am sure I made the right decision. Probably. Hopefully.

Raj, a friend of a friend of Neil, who's an old friend of Howard's, calls from the lobby. I go down to meet him, not thinking how difficult it might be for me to identify an Indian stranger in the lobby of a Delhi hospital. When I step out of the elevator in the lobby, Sanjiv is standing there, as if I'd called for him. He helps me find Raj in a second lobby on the first floor.

We know we don't have the luxury of time to act like strangers. We hug. He asks about Howard. I confide to him all my fears and what a traumatic morning it has been. Raj says we are welcome to stay at his house when Howard is released. "Tomorrow, I bring you a mobile phone and phone card so you can call home." He refuses to take any money for these gifts. "You are friend of Neil's," he says. "You are in my country."

And that is enough. I am in a country of very generous people. I am a guest, and I'm being treated like a royal one.

Two o'clock comes slowly and leaves quickly. Still no word about Howard. I'm not going to be the waiting fool. I need someone to tell me what's going on. By 4:30 I call Sanjiv. "Dr. Trehan said they would be finished by 2:00," I say. "Please find out if something is wrong."

He promises to call me right back. "Do not worry. God will take care of him."

While I wait, I imagine the doctors plotting to keep their mistake from the press. They are probably arguing about who should tell me that something has gone terribly wrong, knowing the world is watching. I think of Alan, Howard's son. Suddenly I'm more afraid than I was this morning. How could I ever tell Alan that his father died in surgery? I remember my father describing his last job in the Army. He had to fly accompanying dead soldiers in their body bags, and then inform their families they'd just lost their son or husband.

And what about me? Howard is the man who made it possible for me to love again. I do not want to lose him. I do not want to fly home with him in the cargo compartment. I will not go home without him. Period. I also do not want Howard to suffer or be frightened. I stare at the phone. Call. Please call me.

Another hour and a half of staring at rickshaws and motorbikes out the window, praying, crying, and finally the phone rings. It is 6:00 and Sanjiv says Dr. Trehan wants to see me in his office.

Sanjiv escorts me first to Recovery to see Howard. I'm surprised that my message has been passed along. I am getting what I asked for: to see Howard as soon after surgery as possible, and to have Dr. Trehan talk to me.

In Recovery, another doctor tells me the surgery went well. They went in through his right ribs and replaced his valve with a tissue valve. So Howard got his pig valve! When I look at Howard, he seems fragile, untouchable. It will be a while before Howard knows I am here, and Sanjiv says we must go to Dr. Trehan's office now.

We sit in the outer chambers until Dr. Trehan asks for me. This time, he remains standing. "Everything went well," he says. "The risk of two surgeries in a row is with the heart muscle itself, and Howard's heart is fine."

I can feel a knot inside my stomach loosen. I look more deeply into the eyes of this man standing before me. I hope he feels my gratitude. I hope he understands that I know he is as tired as I am.

Sanjiv delivers me back to my room and orders my dinner. I try to eat, then call Recovery. The doctor on duty does not want me to visit. I persist. When he agrees to let me come down, he says he doesn't want me to speak to Howard because it might add stress to his heart.

"You may think that, but I do not agree," I say. "I promised Howard I would be there when he woke up, and I need to be there."

When I get to Recovery, the same doctor walks over to Howard's bed. I imagine he intends to block me from getting close enough to speak to Howard. Instead, he gently shakes Howard's shoulder to wake him, then tells me to speak to him.

I can only guess what Dr. Trehan has told this doctor. But I am glad they are respecting my wishes. I can't believe for a second that seeing someone who loves you when you wake up from surgery—instead of a stranger—would add more stress to your heart.

"I am right here, Howard," I whisper. "Just rest and I will see you in the morning. I love you."

Thursday, September 30, 2004

I wake from a nightmare where my best friend, Susan, came busting through my front door, screaming at me that I'm a selfish bitch, I never do enough for her. In the dream I was tired from staying up all night, finishing a painting for her birthday. I showed her the painting and she hated it. My face and pillow are wet. I feel exhausted even before I get off the sofa. My eyes are puffy from crying.

At 7:00 A.M. I call Recovery for a report. "He is improving gradually," the doctor says.

"Is he awake?" I ask.

"Yes, he is awake. You may see him at noon."

I tell him I must come earlier, and finally he says I can come at 9:00.

Evidently the word is out that this American is not going to follow visiting hours. I wonder who I can ask what the Hindi word for "bitch" is, so I will recognize it if I hear it.

Medha arrives from Information with five choices of hotels where Howard can recover when he is discharged. I keep thinking of Raj's offer, and hope I can make a decision without offending everyone involved. Who knows what is offensive? Or how many questions I can comfortably ask? I wish someone could tell me.

Sumitra, one of the sisters in a brown uniform who stops by my room more frequently than any of the sisters, comes in to say good morning. She has become accustomed to seeing me first thing, and also stops by to say good-bye before she leaves. I have learned that she has a son named Jason, and (if I understand correctly) that her husband is sick and doesn't work.

One day she motioned out the window to where she catches her bus to go home, and I watched the way Howard had watched me, until I could see her down on the street and wave to her.

I raise my hands to my forehead and say, "Namaste." She seems pleased to hear the greeting. I continue, "Sumitra, how do you say 'I am sorry' in Hindi?" She looks puzzled. I walk past her and pretend to bump into her accidentally. "Oh, sorry," I say. "Now, how do I say it in Hindi?"

Sumitra smiles. She understands what I need to know. As do I! I keep bumping into people in the hallways and elevators, and can only mumble "Sorry." I find myself wanting to apologize for troubling the sisters, but have no words.

"'Maph karna,'" she says. I hand her my little notepad and pen, and she writes the phrase "'Maph karna.'" Sumitra teaches me a few more Hindi words, and writes them down for me.

Dhanyawaad means thank you. *Kal malenge* means see you tomorrow. *Thek hai* is fine or okay or all good. It is the word all the sisters say when they toggle their heads in agreement. I ask Sumitra about her teenage son, Jason, and she tells me he took an exam yesterday. She is pleased that I remember Jason's name. She makes me feel very well cared for, and in a different way than by Sanjiv or Naruna, who I'm sure have been charged with meeting my needs. Sumitra probably isn't even supposed to be talking to me personally.

When she leaves, I eat breakfast. Then I make a poster of new Hindi phrases. "Maph karna" goes into the center, in bright blue marker.

Sumitra returns with another sister named Bindi. Both women wear brown instead of white uniforms, which I assume signifies a nurse's aide instead of a registered nurse. Sisters. I must remember all nurses are called "sisters." And it has nothing to do with Catholicism. I ask what Bindi's name means in Hindi, and she points to the maroon dot on her forehead at the bridge of her nose, between her eyes.

"And you are sure it does not mean you are married?" I ask.

They both giggle. "It is like jewelry," Bindi says. She takes off her dot and sticks it on my forehead. I point to indicate that it matches my pants. We all laugh.

I show Sumitra and Bindi the chart of Hindi words. "Sumitra is teaching me Hindi," I say. Everything makes us laugh. And I *really* need to laugh right now.

A sister brings me a newspaper, the *Times of India*, which has a headline story about Howard coming to India. I check my e-mail. Jackie, my Web designer who set up the Web site www.howardsheart.com, writes that since the article came out, there have been more than 25,000 hits on www.howards heart.com.

The whole world is watching, and people from everywhere write to us. Some are Indians living in America, congratulating us for our trust in Indian doctors. Some are patients with similar diagnoses to Howard's, who want to know if they should go to India too. Many are from people right here in India, their cities completely unfamiliar to me, offering their prayers for Howard. And reporters—from every television, radio, and print media—all wanting to interview Howard. Yeah, right. Take a ticket, get in line! I will be the first to interview him.

Just before 9:00 I start my journey to Recovery. The guards say nothing but smile when I greet them with "Namaste." The doctors are still making rounds when I enter Recovery, and several sisters are positioned around Howard, intent on whatever they are doing to him. He seems to be thrashing. I see an arm go up. The sisters try to hold him down. He must be in terrible pain. But he's moving. Such a change from yesterday's anesthetized state. I wait at the door until a sister waves me to come to his bed.

"He is slightly agitated," one sister says.

"We give him more sedation." Another sister injects the contents of a syringe into Howard's IV. At home, I would ask the name of the sedative, but I am shocked by the change in him. "Wild." "Combative." I think that's what patients on the psych ward are called when they act like this.

"He has slight fever." I realize it's because of his fever that they have covered Howard's naked body with ice blankets, like giant ice-cube trays wrapped in light blue plastic. It seems very strange to see his bare skin, so taut and pale under the ice cover. "He soon is calm," the sister says. "Is not good when patient is so agitated."

"No, of course not," I say to no one in particular. But I feel that clutch in my stomach. The sisters have their hands full, and, instinctively, I know I should leave them to get Howard under control.

I am only in our room long enough to watch the lemon-lime birds flying in and out of the trees just below my window. All I can do is follow their short flights like stitches among the leaves. It is a rhythm like breathing. I remember the meditation of following your breath. Inhale, exhale, inhale, exhale. I fight off flashes of Howard's arms flailing. I must find out the name of these birds.

The phone rings. Dr. Mehta, the Head of Anesthesiology, wants to see me. Rita, the nursing supervisor, comes to take me downstairs to his office. First, we stop by Recovery, and Dr. Mehta is standing by Howard's bed with another Indian man in shirt and tie, no white coat. They each shake my hand and introduce themselves, but their words evaporate before they reach me.

I am looking at Howard. His eyes are closed. He is much calmer now. I walk over to his side and lean down. He seems so exposed under this ice blanket, which can't be more than two feet by three feet. (Of course, Howard would correct me with the exact number of inches, just by sight.) I want to cover him. That instinct surprises me, since I've never been known for my modesty. But Howard is lying here naked under an icy cover with dozens of people milling about him. It just doesn't seem right.

"Howard, I'm here. You're doing fine." He opens his eyes for a second, and I know he hears me. And I do not upset him! I desperately want to think of something new to say. But it's not like I can tell him about the book I'm reading or a movie I just saw—I am suddenly aware of how he has taken up all the space in my current world; every speck of time, every dab of energy, every thought. "Just hang on, baby. All you have to do is rest now." I reach over the side rail and try to find a clear path to touch him.

Tubes sprout from everywhere: in his hand, his neck, an IV in his other arm, and that plastic vacuum hose still coming out of his mouth. His hair is matted around his face, but I touch his forehead. I'm sure he would ask me to brush his hair if he could talk. I find a space on his upper arm to press two fingers against. He is freezing cold! I pull my hand away. He's not even clammy. He is icy! I want to wrap him up in me, but I cannot even hold his hands. They are swollen and pale with cold.

"We must control the fever." I look up to the sister who is taking care of him. "Do not worry."

I nod. Sure. Easy. Just don't worry. "What is the fever from?" I ask. "The surgery?"

"We do not know yet," the sister says. "But it is normal."

Normal? Fevers are not normal. They are the opposite of normal. They are a sign of infection; that much I know for sure. What else? Two surgeries, back-to-back?

"Please come with us now?" Dr. Mehta asks.

I try to remember how to be polite. "Yes, of course. I'm sorry." I look at the man next to him, extend my hand again. "I'm Maggi. I've already forgotten your name. Sorry."

"Not a problem," he says. "I'm Sakti Srivastava. We have e-mailed a few times...."

"Dr. Srivastava!" I say. "I am so embarrassed. I didn't recognize your name. I was so worried about Howard." This gentle man is my son Bryan's professor from Stanford.

"I understand," he says. "Howard has been through a lot, I hear." His English is perfect, no accent at all. His eyes are clear, his smile is warm, and his voice makes me take a deep breath, as if he were family coming to help me.

"I'm so glad you are here. It is so nice of you to come."

"Let's talk in my office," Dr. Mehta says.

Sister Rita is still waiting for me, and we all follow through another maze of doors.

When we get to Dr. Mehta's office, Rita waves me on. The two doctors and I go in to sit down. Dr. Srivastava has already been told about Howard's two surgeries. But in the way old friends tell stories of things they have done together in the past, Dr. Srivastava and I catch up to this, our first face-to-face meeting, reviewing how we came to know of each other (as if for Dr. Mehta's benefit).

Since the day I lay shivering on my parents' love seat, Dr. Srivastava is the closest thing to home I've felt in the entire week. I know instinctively why Bryan trusted his opinion so completely. He and I sit and talk for a long time about regular things: about his dream of creating an exchange so that U.S. citizens could come easily to India for health care; about his Stanford medical students being exposed, firsthand, to the differences in health care around the world; about living in the same apartment complex as my son Bryan. Someone in India knows Bryan! He tells me how he came to recommend Escorts and Dr. Trehan to us.

"I have talked with other people who have been curious about the option of coming to India for treatment, but no one has followed through," he says. "You are brave to have done all you needed to do to make this happen. I can tell you are an organizer."

And I'm thinking that this kind man, a total stranger until this moment, is the one who made it possible for us to be here. We talk about what made getting to India so difficult. We agree the answer is what my father says is always the answer: communication.

"I found out the Escorts Web site has the wrong phone number on it," I say. "The country added a number, but the Web site had not been updated. I was so frustrated."

"Technology is superb among the Indian people, but the response time is very different," Dr. Srivastava says.

I nod. "I could not get anyone from Escorts to e-mail me back, until you stepped in." We talk about how to improve this because once we arrived, things moved quickly. Howard would still be in Durham waiting for his pre-surgery tests, had we stayed home. "But time here ..." I struggle with what is still an unformed sense I have about time. "I keep getting the idea that we don't have the same concept of time as these people. I don't know what it is exactly—it's as if the words "now," and "next," and "then" mean something entirely different here."

"That's interesting that you noticed," Dr. Srivastava says. "Time, in the Hindu belief system, is not linear, but circular." I try to picture this. Each notion of time I can think of is linear: the time line in a history book, the life lines in your palm. Dr. Srivastava continues, "At any moment, time may look linear, straight in front of you, but that moment is a point on a circle."

I picture a geometry class, where a tiny segment of a circle, taken alone, can look like a piece of a straight line because its curve is so slight. I think about this carefully. If time is circular, and we travel the circumference, then we never really leave anything behind. It accounts for the carpe diem philosophy (enjoy the pleasures of the moment without concern for the future), the live-in-the-moment, it-is-not-the-destination-but-the-journey-that-counts, and you-never-really-arrive concepts.

Time has no beginning, no end. You start when you finish. Nothing is exclusively in the past or the future for we return to everything and incorporate it all like a rolling snowball. If we look at the sacred spiral as a circle sprung loose, we still carry the past inside us, often trying to bury it as we live.

Dr. Mehta goes in and out while we are engrossed in conversation. Finally, Dr. Srivastava must leave for another appointment. He promises to come back. I hug him. He opens the door, and Sister Rita is standing in the hallway, waiting for me.

"Your lunch is getting cold," she says. Her eyes glitter even in this basement light. If she has become tired of standing there, I am the last to see the signs. But something tells me she is enjoying this license to watch over me, wherever it has come from.

After lunch, I fall asleep on my black sofa until the phone startles me awake. "You see Mr. Howard now?" asks a mild voice.

"I'll be right down," I say, and slip into the rubber sandals.

When I speak to Howard, he opens his eyes with a yearning I've never before seen in him. He tries to speak, but the ventilator makes sure no words can come out. I rub the one place on his arm I can get to, touch his fingers. If I had not just seen his eyes I might think he'd died while I was upstairs. He is so cold. I look up at the monitor above his head. His temperature is 38.4, and I try to recall if 36 or 37 degrees centigrade is normal. I know the ice blanket is necessary, but it seems so brutal.

"Squeeze my hand if you love me as much as I love you," I say. I lay my fingers within his reach, trying not to disturb anything that's hooked up to Howard. He squeezes hard, first with one hand, then the other. He blinks. I resist the idea of communicating with Howard by number of blinks, as

I have seen in too many movies about spinal cord injuries. "I got an e-mail from Alan. He's doing fine at his friend's house," I say. "And Norman painted the steps to your house and is checking on the cats." Howard blinks.

Dr. Gaya, the first woman cardiac surgeon I have seen here, comes to the end of the bed.

"Please," I say, "what medications is Howard on now?"

She explains to me that he is on two different drugs to stabilize him, one for heart rate and blood pressure and one for pain. "We are reducing ventilator support, and he is beginning to take breaths on his own in between," she says. "He still has a slight fever, so we keep the ice on him."

"And do you know what is causing the fever?" I ask, hoping against the obvious.

She looks down. "The fever is of some concern. It could be caused from going in the same port for the two surgeries, or it could be fluid collecting in his right lung." She is professional but I see the compassion in her eyes. "We are trying to get that fluid out and keep it out. And we changed antibiotics this afternoon to a full spectrum."

I remember a friend who fell into a coma after wrapping his car around a tree. I sat with him overnight in the hospital, watching him, sucking the secretions out of his tracheotomy, watching the respiratory therapists come in to try to get him to expel the fluid in his lungs. His temperature was raging from the infection in his lungs.

"We are growing cultures of his blood and sputum," Dr. Gaya says. "And we will not try to wean him from the ventilator too soon. It puts too much stress on his heart."

I cannot think of any more questions. She is thorough. I wonder if she senses or anticipates my anxiety. "Thank you," I say. "And I'm glad to see a woman surgeon." She smiles and turns to the next bed.

Howard's feet are scrunched up against the end of the bed. I ask the sister if we can move him up higher. "He looks uncomfortable," I say. Then I realize Howard's 5 foot 11 inches is tall compared to many Indian men. These beds just aren't made for Americans. I take each foot in my hands and gently massage it. It is like holding a frozen roast. His feet almost blend in with the sheet beneath him. When I say good-bye to him, his forehead is burning up. I think of Frost's famous poem *Fire and Ice*. "Some say the world will end in fire, / Some say in ice...."

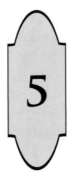

5

LITTLE BROWN BUGS

Friday, October 1, 2004

It is October when I wake the next morning. Never did I think I would flip the calendar without Howard here. I call Recovery. Howard is stable, but there is no improvement. He is still on the ventilator, still has a fever. They tell me I may come at noon. I ignore this, knowing each day I must reassert myself and show these people I am not a visitor from Delhi stopping by on my lunch hour.

I make an altar in a small alcove in the wall near the door to our room. I tape up the mandalas we made, the card that has come from Dr. Srivastava and his family. I arrange all the good luck pieces our friends gave us at home: a pink quartz heart from Sarina, a pewter heart from Molly, Susan's two ivory angels and a worry stone, the metal leaves that Pat made. I take the worry stone and put it in my pocket. I decide to create another mandala.

My intention comes quickly and clearly this time: to get any infection out of his lungs, so the fever will go away. I draw a circle on a clean sheet of paper. I begin drawing little brown bugs of all shapes marching away from the center of the circle. I get only the direction of the bug stampede established before the phone rings.

"His fever is almost gone." The sister in Recovery sounds matter of fact. I do not think I can adequately explain about the mandala and my prayer, only minutes before, for the infection to leave his body.

"I'll be right down," I say instead.

When I arrive, the sister is standing over him, saying, "Take deep, slow breaths." Howard is sitting up! The ice blanket is gone, and he is covered with one white sheet.

"Good morning, darlin'," I say. I do not want him to catch a whiff of the drama I feel inside. "Do what she tells you, now—deep breaths."

He extends one arm and rubs my face, squeezes my hand. He never did follow other people's instructions very readily. He smoothes the sheet over his right thigh as if he were leveling out sand and draws with one finger. D .. A .. Y .. S

"How many days?" I ask. He nods. "You've been here three days. It's Friday." I try not to look at his face. I don't want to tell him the whole story until he can talk and ask questions. There is so much to tell.

He draws more letters on his thigh. C .. H .. E .. S .. T. This is like the game we used to play, writing secret messages on each other's backs with our finger, letter by letter. But guessing Howard's questions is easier … so far.

"No, they didn't cut into your chest. They went in through the side." He rubs his feet against the railing at the foot of the bed. He is waking up. It must be impossible to smile with a ventilator down your throat, whether it is breathing for you or not, but Howard looks as happy as a person can look hooked to so many medical devices. I check his temperature on the monitor above his bed to make sure it is 37-something.

The sister explains that "suddenly his temperature started going down. This is very good," she says. "But now he must breathe on his own."

Again, Howard will be weaned from the ventilator slowly, hopefully by tomorrow. Then he can resume listening to his tape of O Brother, Where Art Thou? We did not expect two surgeries, but we did know they always go for the repair first if at all possible, then replacement. I tell myself this is okay, as long as he is stable.

The next doctor who comes into Recovery says to me that Howard is doing extremely well. "Now, over the next twenty-four hours or so, we will start taking all the other lines out—the one feeding him, the one giving him extra fluid to ensure his kidneys are functioning well" (which they are).

"I know he will do better in our room where it is quiet," I say. I know Howard wants out of the beep beep, lights-on-all-the-time room. But here he has one sister in charge of him, and she stands over him round-the-clock adjusting and caring for him in a way I never could. Once he is doing everything on his own, then it will be smooth, gradual sailing after that.

I leave so that Howard will breathe with her. When I say good-bye, he waves both hands to me. For the rest of the afternoon, I can't get a tune out of my head—"What a Difference a Day Makes." Then, CNN arrives. One woman reporter and a man with a camcorder.

The reporter interviews me about why we chose India, about the cost of Howard's surgery in the U.S., about any reservations we had about having the surgery done in India. She is familiar with the Web site and wants to film me sitting at the computer at the nurses' station. The photographer stands behind me, and asks me to click on www.howardsheart.com over and over again so the home page opens up, like catching a flower while it blooms, in slow motion. Then he shoots me from the side as I'm typing, presumably sending an updated Howard report to my Web page designer, Jackie, to post.

I must decide if I want to keep my reading glasses on so I can actually see what I'm typing, or take them off and type gibberish that I can't see myself—I don't know what will show in his footage. We interrupt all the activities at the sisters' station, and I feel guilty at the presumption of privilege. I know I'm the only patient using their computer to stay in touch with our family, friends, and as it turns out, the entire world. I remind myself that Escorts must plan on benefiting from our experience, so I just try to be gracious to those we displace.

The woman reporter tells me this initial interview is only a segment of the final program that will air. Today's shoot will be opening footage for a larger story they will do after the press conference with Dr. Trehan. Press conference? For some reason, I am not even fazed by this.

I try to watch CNN, but the news is all about the elections back home. I couldn't be less interested. At six o'clock, I go back down to Recovery—one of the few times I stick to official visiting hours. Howard is sitting up with only an oxygen mask on, no ventilator! I clap, try not to let my eyes even think they will tear up. It is such a relief to see him so awake.

He pulls aside his mask and speaks: "Pretty g-g-g-o-o-o-o-o-o-o-d, huh?"

"You mean they didn't fix your stutter while you were under?" I ask.

He cocks his head and smiles. "None of them would call you a couple of hours ago because I pissed them off." His voice is deep and scratchy.

"What did you do?"

He shakes his head. "I'll tell you later." He darts his eyes to each side of him, as if someone might hear him. I remember we have lots to tell each other, and "later" suits me just fine.

Right now, I see the elastic straps attached to the oxygen mask are digging into Howard's cheeks. By demonstrating on my own imaginary mask, I ask the sister to loosen them. "Do you have a bigger one?" This one looks like a child's mask. She shakes her head, lifts the straps to reposition them. "Maybe we can put some gauze under them so they don't cut into his face like that," I say, wincing at the deep red marks. Again, I wonder if Howard can be that much bigger than any patient from India.

A doctor comes over to look at Howard's chart. I ask him about edema. He explains they are giving him extra fluids to make sure his kidneys keep working. I have a sudden panic. I hadn't even thought of kidney function. But my ex-husband was a kidney transplant surgeon, and no one has to tell me what happens if the kidneys shut down. We'll take the edema—I tell myself it might be the only time Howard doesn't look absolutely skinny to me. "What about pain meds?" I ask the doctor. "How much is he on?"

"A very small dose," he says. "We cannot afford to sedate him too much. He needs to breathe on his own."

The pieces start to come together. Sedation for pain control and agitation also sedates automatic mechanisms like breathing. Tricky stuff, this anesthesia.

"So when will he come back to our room?" I ask.

"We will watch him through the night and assess him again in the morning." The doctor takes a couple of steps backwards. "If he continues to improve, we will start taking all the other lines out."

"What are all the lines for again?" I ask.

"One is feeding him; one is giving him extra fluid to ensure his kidneys are functioning well."

"Which they are, right?" I ask.

He nods. "It will be at least a day or two before he can be moved to your room."

I suggest that Saturday night would be great, but he has already moved on to the next bed. I am sure Howard wants out of this buzzing, brightly lit room.

Howard pulls his mask aside. "I don't think they'll let me till you're not here." I have no idea what this means. I wonder if he told them I could take care of him just as well as the sisters can, or something offensive like that. I guess I'll find out. Howard's hair is braided and pulled tightly into a high ponytail.

Dr. K., the cardiologist, comes in and tells me things are going well. Again, I suggest Saturday night as a perfect homecoming. "There is no surgery on Sundays," he says, "so Howard will get lots of one-on-one care over the weekend."

Once again, I find myself caught in the murkiness between being assertive and compromising Howard's recovery. Too many times over the last few days I've imagined dramatically different circumstances than Howard sitting up in bed, talking (even if he did make everyone angry the minute he spoke). We've avoided the worst so far. But breathing, kidney function, infection—the stakes are still high. I decide to remain grateful instead of practicing assertiveness.

THE WAITING GAME

Saturday, October 2, 2004

I call Recovery at 7:30 A.M. Maya, the sister on "Howard duty," says I can come down. At the elevator, a doctor I don't recognize stands beside me. He speaks to me: "You have not updated the Web site lately."

I look at him. "You read it?"

"Every morning." The elevator door opens and he gets off.

I wonder if Dr. Trehan gathers the medical staff together at 6:00 A.M. for "Grand Web site Rounds" to review what I'm telling the rest of the world about Howard's care here at Escorts. Surely not. But how would this doctor even know about it?

When I step inside Recovery, Howard is slightly elevated in the bed with no oxygen mask. He is still receiving oxygen through his nose, but I can see his mouth!

"For his comfort," Maya says. "He also has one neck line removed." Maya is a kernel of beauty—her tiny hands, her eyes and nose and lips are so delicate, I want to cradle them, so even her own smile will not disturb them. I've started asking the sisters the English meaning of their Hindi names. It's no surprise that hers means "illusion."

A doctor stands at the foot of Howard's bed and says, "Next we will take out the rest of your lines and move you upstairs." I almost hug him, and then remember. I am painfully slow to learn that "next" means that is the next course of action. In this case, it could be in the next two or three days. I try desperately to grasp the notion of the Hindu time wheel. I remind myself that Howard will not remain here in Recovery forever; it is not a place a person stays forever. I think back to when my children were two and still in diapers, and I told myself that they would not go to college in Pampers. In fact, they didn't.

"Something is wrong," Howard says. I look at him, but his face shows no emotion that I can read. He rises up toward me and repeats, "Something is wrong. Everyone around me has gone. Everyone here now came in after I did, and I am still here. Something is wrong." He leans back against the pillow.

Gulp. My eyes sting. I will them to stop tearing. It is time for me to tell him what he has been through. I look to the doctor and Maya and mouth the words, "I tell him now?" The doctor nods and turns away.

I move closer to Howard's head and hold his right hand in mine. "Everything is fine now," I begin, and swallow hard. "But I couldn't tell you the whole story until you were fully awake. You wouldn't have understood." He keeps his head centered, but his eyes are wide open and staring directly at me. I'm on.

I reveal the fact that he needed a second surgery, which Dr. Trehan was, in fact, able to perform successfully; and how his own physiological responses then closed off the blood supply to the rest of his body. I tell him they had to go back in to replace the valve.

"Not because the repair didn't work or wasn't possible," I say. "The operation went well. Your body just didn't agree. So, you had two surgeries, practically back-to-back."

His eyelids, still greasy, close. I continue, "It's no wonder you are tired." I give him a second to digest what I've just told him, and to take a big gotta-sound-optimistic gulp for myself. "So now you have the pig valve we talked about, and it's working fine, so it's just as if they decided they needed to replace it from the start instead of thinking they could repair it, so it's a few days later than you think, but...."

"I pissed off the nurses," he whispers.

"That's what you told me last night," I say. "How could you do that ... already?" I look to Maya for confirmation. She is busy writing in his chart.

"The nurse I had in the night was excellent." He speaks very slowly. "She gave exquisite back rubs. Combed my hair. Braided it."

I nod. "I see your new ponytail. So how did you piss her off?"

"Not her," he says. Each word seems to be an effort. "Then I got a new nurse in the morning who was slow."

"Slow?" I imagine Howard asking her to rub his back faster, or braid faster.

"She would do one thing, then write it down. Then another, and write for ten minutes. She kept looking things up in a book." He explains how he lost confidence in her. I suggest it is only in contrast to the superior care he's received so far. "I wrote on paper that she was ten times slower. Asked if I could switch."

"You gave that note to her?" I ask.

"No. Waited till the doctor came. Gave it to him. It spread like wildfire," Howard says, each word deliberate, efficient. "Everyone was pissed off. I'm sure they thought, some privileged American asshole."

"What happened to the nurse?" I ask.

"I think she went home. But it created quite a stir."

I look around at the sisters. When they make eye contact with me, I get a variety of responses—from coy grins to rolling eyes to shrugging shoulders—as if they have no idea what Howard has done. One or two sisters giggle and turn away.

I think fast. Remember my own mantra: "You gotta ask for what you want." The sister may have been incompetent, or she may have simply been thorough. She may have a different style than the others, slower, and Howard doesn't do slow. But I know one thing for sure. Howard must feel confident in this care if he is going to cooperate with them.

I know him well enough to imagine him thinking he can take care of himself just fine, and up and leaving. I also know that a big part of caring for people who feel helpless is to find ways, even tiny ways, they can feel in control. That was how I parented my children, and how I learned to help my aunt after her strokes, a friend during chemotherapy, and my painting teacher in her last days with Hospice care, at home.

I hope this is the biggest scene Howard will need to make to feel that he is consenting to his care. It is essential that he cooperates.

Maya tells me Howard has been drinking water today. "Now he takes tea."

I lean down to speak close to her ear. "I am sorry for any problem Howard made." I feel twice or three times her size, and she is so delicate so exquisite, I feel like whispering. "Maph karna," I say.

"No problem," Maya says. "He is good patient." She looks sincere.

I look around. Some of the sisters are smiling more than seems appropriate for adjusting the flow of an IV or for writing in their patients' charts. I feel like the only one who doesn't get the joke, but these young women are too professional, too dignified to engage me in any complaint they may have about Howard's behavior. I must let it go.

Howard asks me to bring his book and his Discman to him, though he doesn't seem strong enough to hold a book to read. Maya explains they do not allow books in Recovery. I keep asking anyone who passes by and finally get permission to bring down his Discman, but no books. On my trip to our room, I count the days again. Howard has been in Recovery (which I remind myself is less like what we think of as the Recovery Room and more like our intensive care unit [ICU]) since the first surgery on Tuesday. Five days.

I replay Dr. Engel's charge to me: "Maggi, you get him up right away. The day after. Make him walk the day after surgery, no matter what they say." But how can I when he is tied to IV lines and in Recovery? Maybe they are keeping the lines in so I won't think he is well enough to move upstairs. I don't want the reason he is not in our room to be because it is more convenient for all the doctors to see him in Recovery, or because he is the first American.

I also do not want to insist on something that increases his risks. I do the math again. Two to three days for this surgery, a total of five to seven in the hospital. Even if we begin with Wednesday's surgery and forget Tuesday's altogether, Howard should be back in the room by now. Howard is bored. I think we could manage in our room together. It is why I am here. It is silly for me to sit in the room all day long and let Recovery sisters serve him tea. I must talk to Naruna and Sanjiv.

When I arrive at our room, the private nurse of a patient across the hall steps out to place a new bindhi in my hand. A gift, this one shaped like a thermometer. I peel off the one I have on my forehead and ask her to position the new one. We talk for a few minutes, and I learn that she is on duty with her patient all night and all day long. She has been hired by the family to watch this ninety-something-year-old woman who is in a coma. I get the sense that she would talk to me for the next twenty-four hours if I stood here. She has nothing else to do. I thank her for the bindhi and return to my room where my breakfast is waiting.

Sister Bindi comes in with a package of scarlet bindhis. They are red velvet or felt, round, square, some plain, some with rhinestones. I offer her one but she backs up and smiles self-consciously. "For you."

The Head of Anesthesiology calls for me to return to Recovery. I grab the Discman and a couple of Howard's CDs, and the card I made, which is signed by all the sisters and staff. I try to nest it all close to me so it doesn't seem as though I'm carrying in anything they might need to confiscate.

Dr. Mehta is standing at the foot of Howard's bed with a pool of doctors and sisters around him. "We will move Mr. Howard to another room," he says to me, "a brighter room with a TV, where you can be with him more."

I look at Howard. "Not upstairs to our room?" I ask.

"No, not yet," Dr. Mehta says, his hands in the pockets of his white coat. "We will move him to a step-down ICU room where he will still have a sister with him all the time. First, we will remove all the lines and chest tubes."

"Are these chest tubes draining the entry site?" I ask.

He nods. "We will take them out."

This is the most recognizable step yet for getting Howard back to normal. I'm ecstatic.

"Thank you so much," I say, and nod my way around the whole team surrounding Howard's bed. I look at Howard, wondering what will ever make him smile again if this doesn't.

"That's great news!" I tell him, and walk over to kiss him on his cheek, which is covered with five days of new speckled beard. I've never seen him with a beard before. Howard nods at me, and closes his eyes. Even that little nod seems like a lot of work. I watch the team start to break up, and fear they will ask me to leave now. So, remembering my father's philosophy of "it's easier to get forgiveness than permission," I quickly hold up the card that says, "Howard, Come Home to 4th Floor." If anyone gets upset that I brought it inside Recovery, at least Howard's seen it. I'm relieved when no one objects.

Howard looks at the pink and yellow heart on the front, and I open it to all the signatures inside—the sisters, the food and beverage servers, the cleaning men, Naruna and Sanjiv, and even a few doctors I nabbed in the hallway. One person wrote, "Hurry back, we must party!" I learn what it takes to make Howard smile.

The promise of Howard getting out of Recovery gives me permission to get myself out of the hospital. Even though the heat sucks the breath out of me, being outside is as refreshing as that bottle of water the young man poured for me in front of the elevator door the day of Howard's tests. Still amazed at how difficult it can be to figure out what exactly would make me feel good, I take a walk for the first time since Howard's surgery. Previously, if the doctors had called for me, I wouldn't have wanted the sisters to tell them I was out. I was sure they would've assumed I was shopping. Don't all American women shop while their men are in meetings?

I decide I am shopping, actually. I am looking for bindhis of my own to share with the sisters, and I need a new blank book to write in. I am running out of paper and we've only been here a week. I add "wine shop" to my list, still not sure one exists. But I imagine sipping a glass of Cabernet or Shiraz some evening while I sit on the black sofa and watch my street below. Pure decadence. I head in the direction of the Lotus Temple that I've seen every day from my fourth-floor window. The tourist map Sanjiv gave to me refers to it as the B'hai Temple.

Whichever religion claims it, it is a stunning building made of elliptical shapes; a silver and gold blossom. The first time we spotted it, Howard said it looked like a silver orange cut into sections. I can't wait to visit it with Howard. I walk down the street past the end of the hospital, around the corner, and under an overpass. All along the sides of a temple, short sections of fencing peek out between trees and buildings, but they don't signify any sort of boundary any more than the intermittent sidewalks do.

I see through the fencing to camps set up, side by side: blue tarps and clear thin plastic stretched overhead to provide shelter, or at least shade. The plastic ends are somehow tied to rocks and trees—anything to stake out a family's space. I can see cook pots over fires, babies in their mothers' arms or asleep on the dry ground. It still reminds me of a music festival, but this is no Woodstock or Telluride. This is dusty Delhi.

I try not to stare, but I want to be able to accurately describe this scene to Howard, in case he doesn't get to see it for himself. A man is washing his hair with a hose of some kind. I'm not sure where the water comes from but I can imagine the pleasure of getting clean, while living in all of this dust.

I turn a corner, figuring that if I keep turning only to my right, I will eventually get back to Escorts, no matter how many blocks I go, even without knowing any of the street names. A Brahma cow sleeps in the middle of an intersection; crow-sized birds hop along the top of her body; some perch on her head.

As I step into the road, a child, maybe eight or nine years old, crawls out in front of me. She is crippled. She drags herself diagonally across a major intersection. Only a few yards behind, several women follow, carrying twenty- or forty-pound sacks of seed or flour on their heads. Another child, even younger, skips over to me—a boy or girl, I can't tell—wearing only an oversized white shirt, holding out a very large dented can, chattering something to me about pesos.

I think of the little Spanish I know, and then look at this lighter-than-usual child. It doesn't compute. This child's hair looks gray and knotted beyond hope, except for close shearing. His face and shirt are streaked with mud. Like so many people here, his smile seems permanent. I have no grasp of the money yet, and I certainly don't want to open my fanny pack and start hauling out rupees. I shake my head, looking beyond him for the adult who has sent him, the one who is hoping. No one appears to claim this Light Child.

"No, I have no money," I say, shaking my head to discourage this begging child. He giggles and hops around me. I try to walk straight ahead without pausing, which is difficult with the child circling me, especially when a direction such as "straight ahead" is ambiguous at best, with the street so cluttered with animals, people, and vehicles. Everywhere, rickshaw drivers are leaning out of their open doors, beckoning me to climb in.

After walking so freely back home, the constant need to decline offers of rides is a weighty burden. In the States, people assume pedestrians walk by choice, for exercise; even in an unexpected downpour, no one stops to give you a ride. But I am in New Friends Colony, one of the nicer neighborhoods in Delhi, Sanjiv told me, where some of the Escorts doctors live. It is close by, I can say that much.

I come upon a temple or mosque (I haven't learned how to differentiate between them) that is right next to a park. I am tempted to enter the temple, but I do not know the etiquette and am sure, at least, that I am not dressed appropriately. The park is fenced in and quite large—not just a neighborhood pocket park. Big and little kids are playing some sort of baseball or cricket with a stick for a bat. Inside, I spot a crumbling stone wall to sit on. As I make my way over to it, I feel all the eyes on me. Children in the park, men on the street, vendors parked outside the fence. I'm too self-conscious to rest. I try to look deliberate but relaxed in my stride, circling back around when I don't see any other way out but the opening in the fence near the temple.

The light-skinned child who was begging on the street has followed me inside the park, but now, there are other children, all darker and healthier looking, running toward me from every direction. I feel like a magnet—a Pied Piper of sorts. The Light Child looks so different from all the others.

It is like looking at a shot of Annie in the hit show of that name, her red hair like a beacon, identifying her as the star while all the other children appear in black and white. The children gather around me—all ages, all boys, except for one little girl, maybe four years old, who wears only underpants. One boy tells me not to give the begging child any money. Then he says, "What time is it?"

I look at my watch and say, "It is two-thirty."

A wave of giggles spreads through them. Instantly, I recognize the game. These children are practicing what they learn in school. I remember the call and response of Spanish class: "Mi llamo Maggi" and "¿Cómo se llama?"

"My name is Maggi," I say to the leader. "What is your name?"

More giggles. They recognize the words.

The leader looks intent and says, "My name is Asha." The group applauds. While they squirm and laugh they subconsciously align themselves like the von Trapp Family Singers. More and more children run over a dirt mound and join the audience. I guess there must be nineteen or twenty of them.

I look at the next child and say, "My name is Maggi. What is your name?"

Asha steps out of line and says, "His name is Ros."

I wag my finger. "No. I am asking Ros," and I repeat my question to him. But Ros does not answer. I move on to the next child, and on and on to give each kid a chance to practice. Some answer for themselves and wriggle back into line; others are too shy and allow someone else to say their name. Their teachers would be proud. I hope one of them remembers to mention this day.

I look over at the Light Child still hopping around, still amused, but excluded from this group of school-goers. I see now he has no pants on, only a man's long-sleeved white shirt, inside-out with the label showing in the back. It could be from any thrift shop in America. I wonder if he's ever been inside a classroom.

A group of older boys leaves their ball game and comes over, walking instead of running, acting less eager, more cool, but just as intrigued by my presence in their park. The younger children disperse.

"You like Delhi?" one boy asks.

How can I possibly explain how much I like Delhi? "My husband came to India to get a new heart," I say, pointing in the direction of the hospital. He is not my husband, he did not get a new heart, but it seems the simplest way to go. "I love Delhi!" I put my hand over my heart, and they laugh.

"Now he is in hospital?" another boy asks. He does not laugh.

The older boys' English is much better. I nod. "Yes, and he is going to be all right."

They look at each other, testing whether or not they understand. Then they repeat, "All right! He is good. Yes?" A boy holding a soccer ball bounces it in the dirt.

"Yes," I say, and watch their smiles return. "You do not have school?" I ask, then quickly remember it is the weekend. "Of course, it is Saturday."

The first boy says, "Saturday we go to school. Today is Mahatma Gandhi's birthday. You know Mr. Gandhi?"

I nod. "Yes, of course. So you are on holiday?"

They all nod. The boy with the ball bounces it.

"So that is why so many children are playing today?" I ask.

"Yes."

"I must go to my husband now," I say, wondering if they'll ask me for money before I get away. But no one does. My temporary foray into this other world comes to an abrupt halt. Howard is in the ICU. I turn to leave and all the children follow me to the street. As I walk to the far end of the park and turn the corner toward Escorts, Asha's group of younger children follows me on the inside of the park fence, waving and repeating their names so I won't forget them. And how could I forget these children? One by one they leave the flock and return to their games, as if they know all too much about fading loyalty. The Light Child returns to the busy intersection where the cows sleep in the street. I return to the guard at the gate who waves me inside.

"Namaste," I say.

I am too filthy to be close to Howard. I hurry to our room and shower quickly, throw all the clothes I've been wearing into one of the buckets. I put on my other pair of black pants, the other white blouse, and the pair of white rubber sandals that mysteriously appeared in my room, and return to Recovery. A sister stops in the hallway while I am putting on my mask.

"Mr. Howard is shifted." She points to a different set of double doors marked ICU. "Here. Bed one," she says.

Hurray! Howard has been moved to ICU. All I need to do is go outside to make things start happening.

I tie my mask on and push open the doors. Howard is the first person I see. He is sitting up in the bed in the first room, a real window of real daylight behind him. "Hi," he says with his new frog voice. He emits light with his accomplishment, as if he alone had moved himself to this new room.

"Look at you," I say. "I should have left long ago." I hug him, and kiss him on his forehead. "You even got a room with a view." The smudged window looks out onto gray concrete. But at least it looks out. I imagine a squeegee in my hand, ready to clean the window.

"And a TV," Howard says. "They comb my hair and give me massages. I'm getting excellent care!"

It is exhilarating to hear inflections in his voice. We're out of the woods now. "And how about pain?"

He shakes his head. "No pain. Just a little tired."

Tired? I guess so! A sister from the ICU desk comes in and says there is a phone call for me. I follow and take the call.

"Ms. Maggi, this is Sister Deepti. How is Mr. Howard?"

"He is fine, thank you. He just got moved to ICU," I explain. "But, Sister Deepti, I thought you were not here today."

"I am at home," she says. "Today is holiday. Mahatma Gandhi's birthday. My children are on holiday from school. I will pray for Mr. Howard tonight at prayer."

"Oh thank you, Sister Deepti. He is...."

"You take your breakfast?" she interrupts.

"Yes. Yes, I took my breakfast," I say. "Thank you for calling. And thank you for praying for Howard."

"My children pray for Mr. Howard too," she says. "I see you tomorrow."

"Kal malenge," I say.

Sister Deepti laughs. "Yes, Ms. Maggi. Kal malenge."

The head nurse has just called me from her home on her day off. I try to imagine her in jeans and a T-shirt instead of her uniform, but I haven't seen any women in jeans here.

When I return to Howard his head is bent over a tray of food. He looks up. "Dal," he says. Eagerly, I pick up the spoon to feed him, but Howard reaches for it. "I can do it." He grips the spoon, then hauls his hand up above the soup as if the spoon itself weighs more than he can manage. I am too delighted with my wish come true to recognize this longing for independence. Saturday: no more Recovery. Saturday: Dal soup instead of sedation. Saturday: Howard is feeding himself!

About 4:00 P.M., after the respiratory therapist visits, Howard takes his tea. "Coughing is the hardest part," he says with a deep sigh. I've heard many of the patients in Recovery and upstairs, too, coughing up sputum. It appears to be such a violent action.

Respiratory therapists, sisters, and eventually family members paddle the patients' backs with cupped hands. It sounds like children trying to mimic a stampede of horses. Then comes the hacking, wheezing and gagging, the spitting into tissues, and, finally, the gasping from all the effort— sounds that still make me swallow hard and tense up every time.

Often, when I walk down to my room, the sound of the sputum ritual resounds through the full length of the hallway. It reminds me of walking into an animal shelter and starting up a chain of barking dogs. It's a visceral sound of distress, a routine I am reluctant to get used to.

I understand infection results from fluid and phlegm left in the lungs, which is why elderly people die from pneumonia when they've fallen or have become too weak to move around. Unfortunately, understanding the importance of getting rid of sputum and the normalcy of the activity does not make it any less disgusting. And now Howard has joined the masses. So, I learn to paddle Howard's back and pass the tissues.

"Hiccup." The sister looks up from the chart she is writing in. Howard hiccups again and winces. I look at the sister.

"Hiccups are common," she says. She looks at her watch and writes something in his chart.

Howard hiccups throughout the day. A doctor comes, writes in Howard's chart, and leaves. In a few minutes, the sister brings a vial of a thick medicine that looks like melted Vaseline. "Drink," she says. "For hiccups. Hiccups are not good for you."

I cannot decide which looks worse—the way the hiccups jerk Howard's body, or the idea of drinking this stuff that looks like liquid bacon grease. But Howard takes the vial and tips it up, swallowing every drop. I turn my head to gag. The thick goo quiets him, and for this I am grateful.

Doctors stop by, some alone, others in packs. I can't tell what the customary flow is, and what might be excessive traffic, due to Howard's medical condition or nationality. The hiccups return, and the doctors describe exactly what I'd been thinking: the jarring effect of hiccups is not good for Howard's fragile heart. I remember the story of a friend's father who died of hiccups—nothing could stop them, and he died of starvation.

I step outside the curtain to his ICU room while one doctor removes his urinary catheter. It's been five days since Howard peed on his own. He is eager to try. Another doctor comes to take out a different line. Howard seems to be having something done to him constantly. At least now, he can do more than just lie there.

I pass time by noting the details of the room: the edges of the dingy window sealed with duct tape, the blinds pulled up at an odd angle, his bed with a stainless steel crank instead of automatic adjustments like the bed upstairs. The legs of the patient's tray table and the IV pole's base have been painted over and over again with thick, glossy gray paint. It reminds me of the rusted IV pole I salvaged to hang a birdfeeder in my front yard at home. The sisters in ICU wear greens instead of blues, and clear plastic gloves instead of milky latex ones—gloves that don't even come close to fitting their teeny hands. All the water glasses have plastic lids on. I imagine they are to keep out bugs.

Howard wants to use the bathroom.

"You make motion?" the sister asks.

Howard shrugs. "I have to use the toilet."

Because he has not been up yet, they encourage him to use a bedpan first. Howard insists he can go to the real bathroom.

"Not so soon," the sister says.

Howard loses the argument. "Well, then could you all leave me alone?" he asks. He is beginning to sound like himself.

I step outside the curtain again, but the sister stands her post at the foot of Howard's bed.

"Please leave." Howard shoos her away with a wave of his hand. She looks down but stays put.

Finally, she tells me I can come back into the room. Howard complains about having no privacy, and I am not very sympathetic. We're talking about taking a dump. But only two days ago he flailed under an ice blanket with a raging fever, as pale and as naked as a corpse.

"Why don't we try a game of Speed Scrabble?" I say, "well, minus the speed, okay?" I get out the bag of tiles we brought and deal out seven letters each. "Let's just see how it goes."

Howard's first word is "bed," then he adds an "s." Howard, a Scrabble Master, would normally be on words like "cardiac" and "ventricular" by now. I form words like "rupee" and "bindhi." I am playing Scrabble in Hindi. Howard has trouble turning over the tiles, his eyes keep closing.

"We have the rest of our lives to play," I say. "There is no prize for finishing. Just rest. . . ." Before I have scooped up all of the tiles, Howard is asleep. Everything is so exhausting. Even watching him be exhausted is exhausting.

Upstairs, I e-mail a new posting for the Web site announcing Howard's shift to the step-down ICU bed. Naturally, I mention the Scrabble game, since anyone who knows Howard will see this as the truest sign of recovery. I have learned to eat smaller portions of my supper and try not to feel guilty about allowing my membership in the "clean-plate club" to lapse. My parents would be horrified at what I waste.

Afterwards, I return to the ICU. Howard is sitting up looking renewed. I don't ask, but guess that he has managed to make a "motion" one way or another. If he didn't seem so fragile, I might clap.

"Has it rained yet?" he asks. We both look toward the darkening window.

"No, it's been 95 or 97 degrees each day, but no rain." As if the word "rain" was a cue, I suddenly hear a hammering. Parting the slats in the window blinds, I see the eerie arc of streetlights in a downpour at the hospital entrance. It is raining! "You could make a fortune if you could hone that skill of calling down the rain," I say.

Later, when I return to the fourth floor, it is still raining. I look at the sister behind the desk and ask how to say rain in Hindi.

"*Barish,*" she says. I offer my notebook and a pen. She writes, "*Barish ho rahi hai.*"

"All that for rain?" I ask, and try to say the words. "Bareesh ho rahee hah."

"Hai. It is like Hi," she says. "It is raining. Barish ho rahi hai. Try again."

The sisters are all patient with me as I butcher their language right in front of them. And amused, I am sure. I hope. I repeat the phrase and move to the window to look down on

On our first day in India, Howard stands in the window of our fourth floor room at Escorts, above the treetops. He is already hooked up to the portable heart monitor.

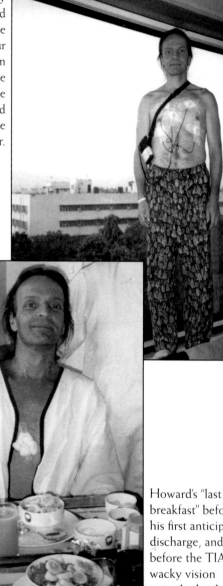

Howard's "last breakfast" before his first anticipated discharge, and before the TIA wacky vision episode that kept us in the hospital for two extra days.

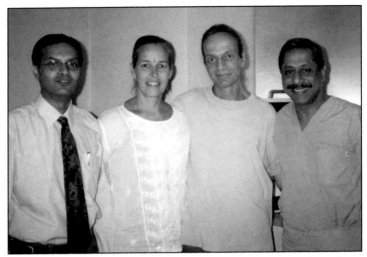

Dr. Satki Srivastava, Maggi, Howard, and Dr. Trehan pose for a farewell shot in Dr. Trehan's office just before discharge to the Centrum Hotel.

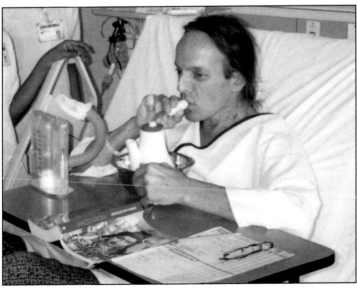

Howard puts down his book to "sip steam" (or as the sisters say, "take steam") from his hospital bed.

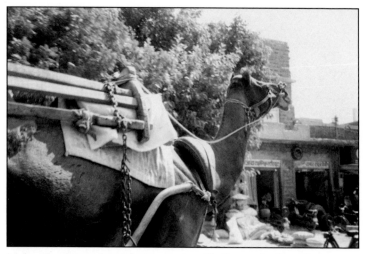

Mahendra drives through the streets of Jodhpur, the Blue City. Maggi's first "up-close" camel!

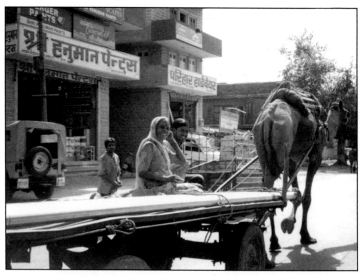

Howard is excited to be able to visit Mahendra's furniture factory in Jodhpur. In India, building materials are transported brick by brick, beam by beam.

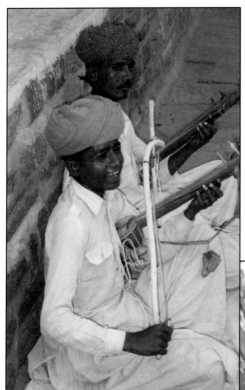

The source of Maggi's "Songs of Angels": Young musicians at Mehrangarh Fort in Jodhpur, Rajasthan, India.

Maggi tours Mehrangarh Fort in Jodhpur, Rajasthan, India.

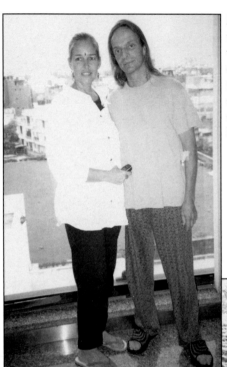

Maggi and Howard stop to rest and look out the west window at the end of the hall on Escorts' fourth floor. The hallway seems much longer after surgery than in the days before.

Howard waits outside the "breakfast room" at our new Jodhpur "oasis" for Mahendra, who is coming to take us sightseeing.

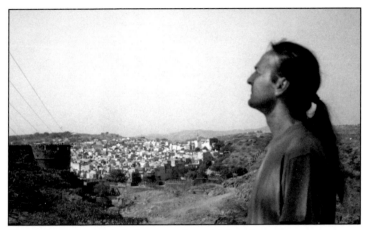

Howard stops outside Lakeview, where Mahendra took us to lunch with the Italian couple, to take in The Blue City, of Jodhpur, Rajasthan, India.

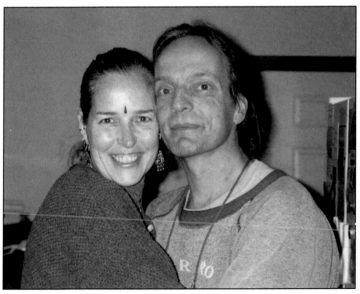

Home again! Maggi and Howard take time out of their new daily routine of Coumadin, walking, sipping steam, and rest to remember how grateful they are that Howard's heart is well, and that together, they face a long life ahead of them.

all of the people walking, some running holding newspapers over their heads, some still pedaling rickshaws.

I imagine those families camped under thin plastic with their babies and cook fires, Brahma cows in the outfield, the crippled children on the steps of the temple.

"What do all these people do when it rains?" I ask the sister.

She looks up from her work, thinks for a minute, then smiles. "It is good to have warm bath, no?"

I suppose it is. "Yes," I say. "Good night. Kal malenge."

From my room, I watch a magical scene—a celebration. I can't bring myself to leave my perch at the window, watching people below still riding their bicycles, walking along the wall at the same pace as if it were noon and sunny, the dark sky flashing like a strobe light above the treetops. I jot down images for a poem so Howard will be able to live this moment too. I don't lie down until the rumbling in my stomach and the thunder have become indistinguishable.

Barish Ho Rahi Hai: It Is Raining

When you woke, tube still in place,
you held up fingers one-by-one
to ask how long you'd been gone
in your curling world of morphine.
In four days of ICU, the streets of Delhi
have mimicked your fever, opposed
your sleep. Tonight you flutter your fingers
asking if it has rained. I shake my head,
try to imagine the dusty roadside camps
in the rain—the children, fires, puppies
and cook pots huddled under torn plastic.
In your room of constant light and alarms,
as if you have called it down, I hear
the rhythm on glass. Barish ho rahi hai.
Upstairs in your empty room, I watch
lightning bathe the dark sky and rooftops.
From this high, streetlights become shower heads,
branches of eucalyptus drip like palms
dipped in silver. But the drenched street remains
dusty, does not reflect like ours at home. Horns
continue their insistence, rickshaws still wind
through traffic, passersby pick up their pace.
Only the buzzards have taken cover.
I ask the sister who comes to say goodnight,
What do people do here when it rains?
She is puzzled, then smiles.
It is good to take warm bath, no?

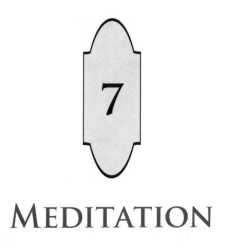

MEDITATION

Sunday, October 3, 2004

In the morning I am weak with fever and chills. Sister Sheela finds me wrapped up on the sofa. "Please tell them I do not want breakfast," I say. I am sure I look as pale as I feel. "Only coffee, please." I take the Imodium my mother insisted I bring with me. Several sisters come by to see if I'm all right. I take Ibuprofen and fear I will etch a path on the floor from the black sofa to the bathroom from all my trips. But I must see Howard. In my whirling mind I contemplate the risk of giving Howard some bug, then realize I probably got it from inside the hospital anyway, or even more likely, that it is just from so much Indian food. It seems risky to stray far from a bathroom, but I dress and make it to ICU.

A sister is paddling Howard's back. He is leaning forward, trying to hack up some sputum. The line in his neck is still in. After she hands a tissue to Howard, the sister tells me his left lung is clear, but he still has a lot to cough up from the right. Again, I think of Dr. Engel telling me to get him up right after surgery. I think, maybe if he got up, he would cough more easily and clear that right lung.

The dietitian comes by, and Howard asks for juice. She tells him he cannot have juice until his blood sugar comes down.

"Would you explain that to me please?" I say. "This is the first time I have heard anything about his blood sugar."

"His blood sugar is slightly elevated," she says. "We are giving him insulin to control it, but until it is within normal range, water is best."

I still don't understand how or why, but decide to wait and ask a doctor. Howard looks at me when the dietitian leaves, he says, "I had no idea I was on insulin."

Two of the surgeons who took Howard into the Operating Room the first time come by, look at his chart, mumble together, then start to leave.

"Uh, excuse me," I say. "With all due respect, please ... I want to understand these issues: the elevated blood sugar, the status of his right lung...."

The tall one turns around to face me. "Well, why don't you tell us the issues you see, and then we'll tell you the real issues?"

He shuts me up. Why I let him, I don't know. Maybe because I want answers before I have to race off to a toilet. I wait. I want information. He explains that Howard's recovery is right on course, that he has no problems. "A postsurgical patient has different signs than a nonsurgical patient.

His blood sugar is well under control. He is recovering on a normal course." He turns back to talk with his colleague.

Of course, he offers no time line, no next step. I am to trust them without questioning—a premise not peculiar to Indian doctors only. That much I know. I have been dismissed before. But during our entire stay, I've heard only one doctor speak in a condescending tone to a sister, during one of the early tests, pre-surgery. Then, I was too new to speak up. Now, I think I would say something. I remember she was one of the smallest, and darkest. I wondered then if she was new too. I saw her tiny wrists and in my mind, compared them to the size of my sons' wrists when they were newborns—hers were tinier, I was sure.

The sister now in charge of Howard gets another sister to help sit him up in a big chair. They have taken out all but one line. He looks frail in the chair. He has lost a lot of weight he didn't have to lose. The color in his face is what we call "prison pallor." From now on, I will associate this pasty gray with hospitals instead of prisons.

One sister brings in a beautiful white urn wrapped in a towel, nested inside a stainless steel tub. "You take steam now," she says. She instructs Howard to suck on the tube inserted near the top of the urn. "Hot steam is good for lungs." I remember back to when my mother spread Vicks VapoRub on my chest when I had a bad cold. She would pin a washcloth under my nightgown to cover the Vicks, and then turn on the vaporizer near the head of my bed. As much as I resisted, it did help.

Upstairs, I e-mail my Web guru again, hoping each bit of good news is received back home with celebration. No need to worry anyone when they can do nothing more than what they are already doing—sending good thoughts to Howard, praying, meditating—whatever they do.

Dr. Echo, the young doctor who wears so many rings, is leaning on the sisters' desk, writing in a chart. Then he edges over toward the computer where I am typing, asks how I am doing.

"It is easier when I understand what is happening," I say, standing beside him. "I was very scared when I did not know what was wrong."

"Of course." I expect Dr. Echo to nod and race off. But instead he puts down the chart and uses his hands to explain again what has happened to Howard's heart. "When a patient is anesthetized, the heart enlarges somewhat—slightly," he says. "The repair of the valve was excellent. But when Mr. Howard began to wake up, his heart, which is small, started shrinking back." He makes the imaginary heart he holds in his hands even smaller. "That's when the long leaflet began obstructing blood flow."

"The opposite of the initial problem, right?" I say.

"Right. The slight leak came later," he says. "Had they waited, it would have been worse. We could have put Mr. Howard on meds after the first surgery...."

"That's what Dr. Trehan said."

"We could have, but because of the physical activity involved in his work, and his bike riding, he could become light-headed, dizzy ... Eventually, well ... he could have been a cripple all his life." Both of Howard's parents were crippled, as he, himself, called them. He grew up accompanying his parents to dances for the handicapped. Crippled, I knew was not something Howard would ever choose. "So the replacement was the right decision," I say.

"Without question," Dr. Echo says. "But I kept thinking about what you both told me the night before the surgery. I admired you then, and was glad we had that discussion. I'm sorry for the confusion."

The night before surgery, Howard and I had walked the halls, trying to make the clock hands spin faster than the sun. We found Dr. Echo at the sisters' station, and spoke to him. "We do not know what your customs are here," Howard said. "But Maggi and I agree that if something goes wrong on the operating table, we do not want you to use extra measures to keep me alive."

Dr. Echo put down the papers he was holding and turned to face us with his full body. "You mean, if your life after that point would be compromised drastically, with irreversible damage, you do not want life support?"

We both nodded.

"I understand," he said. "It is refreshing to hear you say that. So many families do not agree with this philosophy. Thank you for saying so." He shook Howard's hand, then mine, and walked away.

Now, I ask Dr. Echo about my theory that ambulation will help Howard to cough and keep his lungs clear, and also about what feels like quite an extended recovery period from what we'd originally thought. He explains even more. "When a patient has back-to-back surgeries, it is not just twice the recovery period of a single surgery. It is an exponentially greater recovery time due to the increased amounts of sedation."

I nod.

He continues, "The doctors are conservative to avoid any setbacks, dizziness, or other problems." He assures me that the reason I was told to get Howard up out of bed was to avoid blood clots in his legs. "But we are giving him blood thinners to address that."

I am surprised, thinking blood thinners were only for those who receive the mechanical valve.

"Mr. Howard will be on blood thinners for the first three months," Dr. Echo says, anticipating my question, "plus reduced activity. The valve has to seat itself in the body."

"Like a transplanted kidney?" I think of the human body's tendency to reject foreign parts.

"Similar," says Dr. Echo. "I hope you understand that this was a normal complication. It would have happened anywhere."

This is exactly what I have been telling myself and what I plan to tell anyone who tries to suggest the Indian surgeons screwed up. "Oh, I know. I only hope the media does not misconstrue it as a mistake for their story's sake."

"Don't worry about the media," Dr. Echo says. "You have enough to think about."

"I appreciate your talking to me," I say. My first breath after he is gone is deeper and wider than any breath I have taken in the last week. Ten minutes of conversation, of human compassion, and I feel my own heart settling down to rest.

Monday, October 4, 2004

Today, Howard is descended upon in the same way he was the day we arrived at Escorts Heart Institute. Doctors I've never seen before wheel in machines to do more chest X-rays, EKGs, and take out his last line. The sisters have warned me that today is the day; however, they insist he will not go back to the same room, but to the third floor instead.

Dr. Trehan is in the States, so it is Dr. Mehta, Head of Anesthesiology, who brings a team with him to tell me Howard will be moved upstairs. Even though I've tried to learn not to beg, and never ever to grovel, I do both. "I will be diligent," I say. "I will make sure he blows into the ball tube thing, and takes his steam, and does his exercise, and walks. He will do better if he is with me, I promise. It is why I came."

Finally, Dr. Mehta talks to the sisters and other doctors and by some stroke of brilliance, announces that he will send an ICU sister up to be with Howard in our own room 'round the clock. I recognize this compromise as one that probably violates Escorts' rules of care, but I take it and run with it. Howard says a gravelly "Thank you."

It takes only a few sisters and me to wheel Howard from the ICU to the fourth floor. When the elevator door opens, all the sisters cheer for him. Mabel, the ICU nurse who has been assigned to accompany Howard for the remainder of her shift, is my visual cue for the shuffle we just pulled off. She is clad in greens. I imagine she's had different training, perhaps even a different salary than our fourth-floor sisters in their white or brown uniforms. I wonder, "What have I done?"

But having Howard back in our room again overshadows any guilt I might be able to conjure up for rocking the boat or making anyone else uncomfortable. I am here for Howard. I am certain that he belongs with me in our room. I am the first to get to walk him down the hall, which I'm sure must seem five times the length it was before he left for surgery. But Howard appreciates being upright again.

Some delicate negotiating about sharing tasks goes on between green-Mabel and the fourth-floor sisters. I stay out of it and decide they can work it out themselves. The sisters bring more steam for Howard. He sucks on the tube and allows the hot steam to fill his lungs. He winces but seems to enjoy the comfort it brings.

Green-Mabel gives him another vial of syrup for his hiccups, which insist on returning. The hiccups are Howard's biggest complaint. She washes his hair for the first time, towels it dry while he sits in a chair, then combs and braids it.

Howard is bright purple and green from just below his ear, across his right shoulder, and down to his ribs where the incision, at least the main incision, is. We try to act normal, even though Mabel is sitting on our sofa, my bed. When the sky darkens, Howard is tired enough to want to go to sleep. Mabel quietly leaves while I help him get settled down into bed. When he is asleep, I walk down the hall to e-mail the big news to Jackie to post on the Web site. Howard is back in our room! Mabel is sitting with the fourth-floor sisters, and I am grateful.

About 11:00 P.M., a new sister comes to relieve Mabel. They sit together on the sofa in our room and go over Howard's chart, line by line. It is like listening to my grandmother tell a bedtime story in Czech, her native language, when I was little. The lilt and cadence of words I will never understand is both mysterious and comforting. I am aware this is the first sleep Howard has had without the constant beeping and bright lights of the ICU or Recovery Room. He doesn't seem to notice.

Tuesday, October 5, 2004

Other patients and the sisters have warned me that recovering from heart surgery is a gentle roller coaster—good days and bad days—but all moving forward. Tuesday is a particularly difficult day as Howard discovers his new physical limitations in the same room he left only a week ago where he was doing push-ups on the floor. He remains in bed, his body exhausted simply from healing. The coughing, hiccups, getting up to use the toilet, all drain his reserves of energy.

My parents call our room, eager to hear Howard's voice. I hand him the phone without asking if he wants to take the call. As he tries to speak to them in a normal voice, I see his eyes filling up. Before I am aware enough to prevent it, he drops the phone in his lap and starts to cry. "I just can't." He is crying harder than I have ever seen him cry. I want to just hold him, but my parents are excited to know he is going to be fine. I grab the phone.

"He's awfully tired. Sorry," I say. "We'll try to talk to you later, okay?" I wish I had anticipated how emotional this is for Howard. I think post-traumatic stress syndrome—then think, who cares what it's called? He is crying. I just hold him, gently so I don't press too hard on the purple bruises. We rock so slightly, I am sure he can't tell.

Both of my sisters call from Florida, and my son Thane calls from New Zealand. Howard's friend from Iowa calls, and so does his friend from Sweden. I know to ask him before each conversation, but Howard is too tired or too emotional to talk. He is just not ready. Everyone understands. It is Howard's voice they want to hear, not mine. But again, I am clear on who gets what they want this go-round.

The wife of Raj, the friend of the friend of Howard's friend, who offered his home for Howard's recovery, calls on our room telephone. She is in the lobby. She comes up to visit and says she's brought a basket of fruit, but they willl not let her bring it into the hospital. "No food from outside," she says.

She is a lovely woman with warm, friendly eyes. I examine her sari without staring. It is so generous of her to go to the trouble of having her driver bring her here, when she owns and runs a very busy company. I walk her outside to her car, certain I can convince the guard that the fruit is for me, not for Howard. I'm sure he will allow me to bring it inside.

Wrong. Raj's wife gives me a hug, says good-bye, and drives away with the fruit for her own family. These folks are strict. I am glad I didn't get caught smuggling in that Kit Kat bar.

Howard is asleep by the time I get back to our room. I sit on the sofa and watch his chest rise and fall with each breath. It is a comforting rhythm I will never take for granted again.

A strange woman knocks on our door. She comes in, looks at Howard, then introduces herself to me. She is from the American Consulate. I invite her to sit down in the one chair we have, and she pulls it up close to me. In a stage whisper she explains that she has just come from the Consulate.

"Everyone at the Consulate is following Howard's progress. We are watching the Web site and hoping for his quick and full recovery."

"Thank you," I say. "Thank you to everyone." I do not admit that I have no idea what the American Consulate does. Nonetheless, I am pleased that some government officials are keeping Howard on their agenda.

The woman gives me her card. "Please call if you need anything."

The door clicks behind her as she leaves, and Howard wakes up. I assume he might have listened to our conversation but did not want to have to speak himself.

Howard is sweating and keeps asking me to turn down the air conditioner. I turn it down to 16 degrees Celsius, put on as many layers as I can find, and wrap myself in two blankets. We spend our days paddling, coughing, sipping steam, blowing and sucking on the plastic-ball lung game to increase his lung capacity, and walking the halls.

When the sisters come for one more blood sample, Howard is irritable. I decide to let Christine, the current ICU sister on duty, handle this one. The difference between my going to bat for Howard's return to our room versus his not wanting to have more blood work is clear. I don't know how to make peace of this conflict.

Dr. K. invites me to a conference downstairs on meditation. Twice, when I see him in the hallway, he reminds me, and I am quite honored to be included. By 2:00, I leave Howard in the hands of Christine and head to the basement. There is an enormous reception with tables and tables of food in chrome-covered serving platters. I'm not the least bit hungry, but I am happy to see my favorite food and beverage servers in their sparkly teal vests.

The auditorium fills with doctors and sisters and lots of other health care professionals. I take notes when the guest speaker reminds the audience that meditation originated in their culture. We learn to breathe and do a brief meditation that can be used before we start our day, with patients, even when stuck in a traffic jam.

I return to the room excited to tell Howard all about it. He doesn't want to hear it, let alone try any of the techniques I learned. "I just want to get out of here," he says. "They keep poking me, pounding my back, and giving me more medicine to drink. They have enough of my blood. I'm not giving any more." I listen to the faint rumble of a nightmare beginning to form.

8

WE'RE OUT OF HERE?

Wednesday, October 6, 2004

Breakfast comes but Howard is not interested. "You're not going to get stronger by not eating," I say. He gives me that I-don't-need-a-mother look. "I know you don't feel hungry. It's the antibiotics that kill your appetite," I remind him. "But try to think of eating as nutrition instead of as tasty." I cut a rag of his omelet and stuff it between a folded piece of toast. "Just try a bite. Please?"

"I'll try a piece of papaya," he says. I set the sandwich down just as Howard pushes the tray away from him. "I'm going to lie down."

I wish we had a cell phone. But the day I bought a phone card down at the Coffee Shop on the first floor, the hospital changed the entire phone system and I couldn't use that calling card from our room. So, Howard still has not talked to his son, Alan. And, of course, I can't take him out to one of the phone kiosks where they just dial for you, and charge you at the end.

If we had a DVD or VCR to watch movies, the time would go faster. Or at least Howard could multitask and take his steam treatment or do his breathing exercises while he did something else. He is ornery, but I tell myself that, emotionally, he is riding a post-surgical wave of depression. All night long, he was up every thirty to forty minutes to pee. For a lifelong good sleeper and spontaneous napper, this new rhythm has to be exhausting.

I think of my own exhaustion, years ago, when I nursed my babies every two hours round-the-clock. Howard gets exhausted just looking at his lunch. I wash his hair and braid it, but looking good does not seem to make him feel good.

It must be hard on him to have every conversation, every moment of our day, every activity be about his body. He is used to coordinating and supervising his crew, running his household with his son's needs and schedules having top priority. I'm sure this intense focus on himself, especially how he is feeling, is unsettling, at best, and perhaps very disturbing.

I talk with Howard; I acknowledge his freedom to refuse medicine or food. As much as I hope it doesn't come to that, I recognize that his feeling of powerlessness is to be expected. I suggest he make a list of all the medicines he is taking and the specific times he must take them. The sisters know what his meds are and when to give them, so we could gather this information easily. "That way you will know when to expect them," I say. "You will know they will be coming at 2:00 A.M. to give you the antibiotics, and you will know they are on schedule, not just waking you at random to annoy you." Howard doesn't answer.

I curl up on the sofa and work on the poem I began while Howard was downstairs. Sometimes I wonder if he knows how much I care about him, or if I seem like an additional obstacle to his being free. "Want to see the poem?" I ask.

He looks over his glasses. "Sure."

I place the notebook on his bed beside him. "You don't have to read it now."

"Read it to me, will you?" he says. "My eyes are tired."

"It can wait," I say.

"Would you, please?"

And as awkward as it feels, I read aloud to him:

The Wall

All day long empty rickshaws passed, motorbikes
rattled by, with women in saris sitting side-saddle
    behind the drivers
holding babies and newspapers in their laps.
Schoolgirls with plaited hair, brown sox and skirts
walked in pairs; women shared umbrellas
against the sun. I watched the wall below
as if it might crumble before you woke.
Three young men in khaki pants squatted
to paint the wall in patches of stormy gray
that baked to smog before a section was done.
Your heart was already mending, new threads
laced by these Hindu surgeons. And you slept.
Vendors lined up their handcarts of fruit.
Out my window buzzards circled rooftops
and treetops decorated with lemon-lime bee-eaters.

Rickshaws carried loads of brick and pipe
weaving in and out of men strolling hand-in-hand.
A mangy dog sniffed along behind a tractor,
same as yesterday. And you slept.
The doctors called me to your quiet side
with multisyllabic words they had mastered
in English: complications, obstruction—words
to accompany the consent form they held out.
I looked at you, but knew where to sign, returned
to your room to watch the living going on below.
They came to paint the wall again the next day
as if it was not gray enough, as if they had made
a mistake the first time. They painted the same
sections in the same order, saved the corner jog
for the youngest. A man in a red shirt peed there,
in the corner jog. Another and another,
then a student balancing a book on his head
dropped out of step to pee against the wall,
walked on. Young women passed, covering
their mouths with their *dupattas*. And you slept,
eyes greased shut, IVs and necklines
wrapping your head like Medusa's snakes.
The sky darkened, the wall lightened,
and down below, they kept you asleep.

It is difficult to respond to someone else's poem, and I
don't want Howard to feel that he must. So I say, "See what
you missed?"

Fortunately, an unfamiliar doctor, Dr. Gagan, provides a
distraction. He comes in with the head nurse, Leela, and asks

Howard how he is sleeping, if he has any pain, the usual. He listens to Howard's complaint about having to pee all night long, and explains that they have been giving him Lasix, a diuretic, since he was in Recovery to reduce the volume of fluid his heart needs to pump.

"Don't drink anything two hours before bedtime," he suggests. "If you are thirsty during the night, take only sips of water." I then discover Dr. Gagan has not come just to chat, but with the specific mission to remove Howard's cannula, the more or less permanent tube that was inserted into a vein in Howard's left hand as a way to give him medicine intravenously, without having to stick him in a new spot each time. Dr. Gagan removes it and covers it with gauze and tape. One less tube attached. Progress.

Sister Leela and Dr. Gagan turn to leave, but the doctor stops and says, "I will also stop your hiccup medicine unless you think you need it."

Howard shakes his head. "No, I don't. And I don't need any more injections." Luckily, they keep walking out the door.

"Thank you," I call after them.

Another doctor comes to change the dressings on Howard's wounds. We have come to call them "wounds" instead of incisions because they all seem like holes instead of straight cuts—those on either side of his neck, along his right chest, his left groin. His skin is a beautiful combination of purple and green, and his wounds are healing nicely.

While they are exposed, Howard asks me to take photos of each site. He shows me new wounds I didn't even know were there. I don't say it aloud, but I think what a perfect example for my painting students of how to blend two contrasting colors seamlessly, without leaving any straight edges. It feels odd thinking of my own teaching, my students, my art. It's been so long since I've held a paintbrush in my hand. It feels like I've been holding my breath.

While he positions himself and I snap the photos, I can't keep from imagining a sculpture of Jesus with holes in his forehead from the crown of thorns; a hole in his side. I'm glad Howard doesn't have any wounds in the palms of his hands.

A physical therapist arrives and listens to Howard's chest. He says the sound of Howard's breathing is too faint. He needs to be able to hear it better. So he describes some new exercises to add to the list. I take notes, and when he leaves, make a chart.

"Look," I say, when it is finished. "You can mark off the ones you do each time you do them during the day. You don't even have to do them in order, this way." I hope this adds one more activity Howard can be in charge of.

Howard closes his eyes. His despondency accentuates my own fatigue. I have had diarrhea for days, and even messed my sheets last night when Howard was in the bathroom and I had to wait. But I must remain alert, steadfast. I hope this is the bottom point and that things will be better tonight.

I walk down to the sisters' station and roll a chair over to the west window that faces the Lotus Temple. I remember that the Lotus Inn is on the list of guesthouses Medha gave me. It must be over in the direction of the temple. Surely I can find it.

Howard is asleep when I go back to the room, so I change shoes and go out with a new pioneering attitude. My mission is to find our next home. I see the sign for the Lotus Inn after only a couple of blocks. I walk under the freeway overpass and turn west toward the temple where we've watched the sunset stripe the sky in dusty rose, bright orange, and lavender. A motorbike speeds past me at the intersection—it is a

Domino's Pizza delivery guy. Domino's is the pizza company I've boycotted for over fifteen years because of its political bias.

I follow the tall Lotus Inn sign that rises up above the buildings, but I cannot find a way to penetrate the high chain-link fence along the frontage road that borders it. I keep walking. I choose not to ask the construction workers who are shoveling piles of dirt and broken concrete into fabric baskets with thick rolled rims. They remind me of handmade bread baskets. It is so hot; I can't imagine doing physical labor in this heat. They wear flat hats with scarves that fall to cover their necks. Then I watch as one young man lifts a full basket of debris and sets it inside his flat hat to carry it. It fits perfectly. I stop to memorize its design with every intention of one day making a few as a joke for Howard's crew.

I maneuver around several street dogs as I walk along the fence, my window into the campsites staked out behind. They butt up to a secure complex with a sign that says Government of India. I feel this same heaviness when I pass amputees begging in the streets. It is the heaviness that lies in the wide chasm between those who have and will always have, and those who do not have, and never will.

I decide I will let Naruna, the hospitality man who met us at the airport, take me to see the guesthouses. For the moment, I will return to Howard. Even if he doesn't want my help, it is the only place I could possibly make a difference.

Thursday, October 7, 2004

Without turning over I open my eyes and see Howard standing beside his bed smiling at me. He shuffles his feet in a little two-step and says, "Wanna dance?"

"Sure. Can I go to the bathroom first?"

"Yup. But better hurry. I've done all my breathing exercises one time." His voice is still hoarse.

"We don't even get coffee first?" I ask.

"The tray isn't here yet." He opens his arms wide, inviting me to look around the room myself.

By the time I get dressed and fold up my blanket, the coffee and tea tray arrives. I fix our cups and we sit on the sofa together to watch the morning unfold below. I never tire of this blossoming. The fruit vendors roll out their carts, the students in uniforms walk in pairs—one direction in the morning, the opposite in the afternoon—and the birds flit in and out of the trees at eye level. I want to know the names of the fruit. I want to know the names of all the birds and of each tree. Howard is not as familiar with this scene as I am because he spent almost a week downstairs. It still surprises him to see the continuous stream of men who break out of step to pee in the corner of the gray wall.

"Did I tell you they painted that wall twice while you were in Recovery?"

"Why twice?" Howard says.

"I think it's like the Golden Gate Bridge: they just start over when they finish. But everyone avoids the corner," I say. "Both times, a very young boy had to paint the corner."

"Like giving the youngest in the gang the gun," Howard says.

"Now that's a pleasant thought," I say, thinking about the pecking order of men. "But the corner was still wet from the urine."

"How could you tell?" he asks. "Did you go touch it?"

"Yeah." I roll my eyes. "No, it is always darker gray than the rest of the wall, even the newly painted part."

Sakash, my favorite server, knocks and comes in. We exchange greetings, and he exchanges our coffee tray for breakfast. Bread and butter and jam finally show up on Howard's tray. While he prepares his food the way he wants it—banana with his corn flakes, cold milk instead of hot—I ask Sakash the meaning of his first name.

"My name?" he asks, with a smile that is as contagious as anyone's here. I nod. "Sakash is Hindi word for illumination, like lights." No kidding. He must have been born smiling.

"Of course," I say. He nods and turns to leave.

"Today I think Naruna is going to take me to see guesthouses," I tell Howard. "I heard Dr. K. mention one that he likes. But I definitely want to see them before we decide."

"I'm leaving that up to you," he says, pushing the tray away from him. "I'm going to lie down for a minute."

"Want to take a short walk down the hall first?" He is tired, but I know that if he is to get his stamina back, walking is important; also it will help keep his lungs clear. In spite of knowing this, it's still a hard call to push him when he looks so tired. I ask, "Just a short one?"

"Guess I should."

We hold hands and walk to the end of the hall to the long skinny window. The sisters at the desk say good morning. "Namaste," I repeat so many times the word now feels like warm milk in my mouth.

"Okay, let's turn around," Howard says.

I see the computer at the end of the desk is free. "Do you want to e-mail anyone?"

Howard shakes his head. "Later."

We pass other patients walking in their rubber sandals. The paddling and hacking sounds come from several rooms. "Do I sound that bad?" Howard asks.

"Only when you cough up sputum." I let go of his hand and gently rub circles on his back. "It's okay. It's a good-bad sound because it's keeping you from getting an infection."

"It's disgusting," he says. "I'm ready to get out of this place."

"I know you are. I think Dr. Trehan gets back Friday or Saturday." We've been told that Dr. Trehan has been in the U.S. I'll bet anything they won't let Howard go before Dr. Trehan sees him again. My guess is that things will start happening when he gets back.

"I don't need Dr. Trehan to leave here."

Howard decides to change into a T-shirt and a pair of rayon pants. He has grown tired of his "karate uniform." When the barber drops by to see if Howard wants a shave, Howard says yes for the first time. I take a picture. Howard tips him 100 rupees. I hope he isn't secretly preparing to walk out of the hospital. "When he clips my nose hairs, it sounds like an old typewriter," Howard says after the barber leaves.

"Exactly!" I say. "And what's that bar of clear stuff in a glass he rubs on your skin?"

"Antiseptic, I think."

"It looks like some huge uncut diamond," I say.

"Yeah, but a diamond dipped in water," Howard says. "It drips but it feels good."

Friday, October 8, 2004

Everyone comes to check out Howard. They come for one last listen. Sister Rita, the fourth-floor supervisor, has stopped by at least once a day. Today she comes while Howard is eating breakfast. Howard has earned every second of this attention, and I can tell he is ready to celebrate. The discharge papers are being written. A complete set of Howard's records are delivered in a fat pink folder. We will take them to Dr. Engel when we get home.

Howard does his breathing exercises. Naruna arrives to discuss guesthouses he will take me to see this afternoon. I mention that Dr. Srivastava is checking into the Indian International House.

"That is nice but far away," Naruna says. "You must stay close enough to come back here anytime."

Dr. K. has suggested a place called Chanriwal, Diabetes Center and Complex, where an Escorts doctor visits every day. He and Naruna agree Howard could also go to the Escorts Rehabilitation Center, a separate building just in back of the hospital. But Howard is adamant about going to a hotel, not to another hospital. I agree—he needs a complete change of scenery. He needs to feel like a tourist instead of a patient.

A nap, a crossword puzzle, and another meal later, I kiss Howard good-bye, put on my sandals, and meet Naruna in the lobby. While Howard sleeps and waits for all the discharge papers and the last lab work to come back, I will pick out our new home.

"Are you ready?" Naruna asks, his eyes dancing.

Naruna has so much energy, I wonder if he ever gets any sleep at home. During the long days of waiting for Howard to wake up, Naruna and I talked a lot. He told me about his children and about his philosophy of providing opportunities for them. I want so much to meet them; I'm sure they are gorgeous kids.

A driver waits in the Escorts car at the main entrance, doors I haven't seen since the night we arrived. Naruna is obviously knowledgeable and definitely in charge. It's a relief. All I have to say is yes or no. We visit Chanriwal, the Diabetes Center. A man brings a tray of glasses of water for everyone, but when I reach for one, Naruna stops me.

"Bottled water for her," he tells the waitperson. He explains to me that although they are drinking filtered water, it is still not safe for me since I have not been drinking it my entire life. I must drink bottled water only.

The Chanriwal Complex feels like a hospital. I veto it immediately. We visit two other hotels and get the royal treatment at each one. Last stop is the Centrum Hotel, about a mile from Escorts. The manager looks like a young actor with his sunglasses on, and he is every bit as energetic as Naruna. They obviously know each other, and I imagine Escorts has sent patients here before. The manager promises to take good care of Howard. He shows us a room toward the back of the hotel that he assures us will be quiet. But it is dark.

"Do you have a different room with more light?" I ask.

"Only one that overlooks the street," he says. "It is more noisy."

"May I see it, please?" I ask.

To get to the noisy room, we take a small elevator to the second floor over the lobby. It is immaculate. It's spacious with two twin beds (at least that's a step up from a hospital bed and a sofa), a small love seat, a desk, and a huge bathroom with shower. Most of all, a huge picture window overlooking the street. Delhi.

Something clicks inside me, like when you finally find the perfect house and forget to ask how much it costs. "This is the one," I say to Naruna. "We both want to be part of the city. We are on vacation now!"

The manager looks surprised, looks at Naruna for confirmation.

"She wants this one," Naruna says to him. "This includes breakfast for ... what? ... 1,500 rupees per night, yes?"

The manager looks down. "This room is 2,700 rupees." Then he looks at Naruna and says, "Yes, 1,500 for you." They laugh and hug each other. I am positive I don't fully appreciate the price break we just got, but now is not the time to stop trusting Naruna. (I learn later that he negotiated the price down from about $67 to $37 a day, in U.S. dollars.)

"You can hook up a VCR to watch movies?" Naruna asks.

Yes, yes. I had forgotten to ask. Thank you, Naruna, our guardian angel.

"Of course."

"Please arrange for that," Naruna says. "Our driver will bring them later this afternoon."

It is a simple decision. We are moving to the Centrum Hotel. Today. This afternoon.

Satisfied, as the driver approaches Escorts, I ask Naruna if they can drop me outside of the hospital so I can pick up our photos at the shop across the street.

"You want to stop there now?" he asks.

"Yes please," I say. "But just drop me off. I can walk back to the room myself. Thank you so much. I love the Centrum."

"I knew you would," Naruna says. And I jump out in between a swerving rickshaw and a cow. I pick up our photos, reprints I have had made for a collage we plan to make for the sisters. It will be a gigantic card, with pictures of all of them, to say thank you. I resist the urge to look at them before I'm with Howard again. When I arrive at our room, Howard is sitting up in his street clothes, reading. Such a sight!

"I got the photos," I say. Howard just looks at me. "The reprints for the collage."

"But did you get a hotel room?" he asks.

"Oh, yes. A perfect one," I say. "It's called the Centrum. Our room overlooks the street so we can watch Delhi happen close up. It's really clean and big."

"As long as you like it," Howard says.

"But look at these pictures," I say. "Here's the one of you with "dhanyawaad" on your chest. And here's you with Sister Rita."

Howard holds them, moves them even farther away. "I need my glasses," he says. "I can't see them."

When I get up to get his glasses, Howard says, "I've been a little dizzy reading."

I'm excited to see how well these pictures of our Escorts family have turned out and I hand him another photo. But he doesn't take it. Slow response time. After too many seconds, I look up at him. One eyeball is rolled high up in the top outside corner of his left eye and the other has gone directly opposite. His eyes have gone haywire!

"Howard!" I scream. I jump up and hold his face. "Look at me! Howard, look at me!" He cannot see me, I am sure. The movements of his eyes look like roving searchlights.

"Stay here." I run down the hall to the sisters' station. Dr. Echo is behind the desk. "Something is happening to Howard." Dr. Echo drops the chart in his hand and leads a team of sisters to our room. Howard's eyes are still out of control.

Dr. Echo examines Howard, and asks a lot of questions. Howard's eyes return to their normal position. He says he lost his vision except for a small hole. He saw black and white lines, colors, and then his vision returned.

"Now I can see," he says, "sort of."

I am so glad Dr. Echo got to see Howard's eyes moving through their wacky orbits. Not that I'm glad his eyes did that, but I don't want to be the one to convince someone else of what just happened.

Suddenly a young man comes in pushing an empty wheelchair. He announces something to the entire crowd, and everyone makes a path for the chair. Dr. Echo looks at me. "Dr. Trehan wants to see him."

My mind is spinning. I don't even have the ability to question cause and effect here; whether Dr. Trehan has already heard about Howard's eyes, or if his summons is unrelated, coincidental. I follow, which seems like a lot for me to do right now. Someone else pushes Howard in the wheelchair and leads me along until we are presented to Dr. Trehan in his office. Naruna is already here.

Fortunately, Dr. Echo has come with us, and he tells Dr. Trehan about Howard's vision problem. Dr. Trehan examines Howard, asks a few questions, and tells us to return to our room. I learn on the way that we were summoned to Dr. Trehan's office for Howard's final discharge. But just as the wind can suddenly change direction, so does the course of this Friday night.

In a whirlwind, Howard has an ophthalmology consultation, dilation of his eyes for a later follow-up eye exam, a neurological consultation, a CT scan of his brain, and many more pricks for blood. In a murky fog, I try to write down what I can hear and understand. I trail behind the two sisters who wheel Howard downstairs for the CT scan. They take Howard straight in.

I wait in the hallway, then sit next to a man who is waiting. He tells me he is from Bangladesh, and some Crosby, Stills and Nash tune starts playing in my head. No, that was "Marrakech Express." I am ashamed I have no idea where Bangladesh is. He speaks quietly, tells me something about an eighteen-hour train ride from Calcutta, about being here at Escorts twenty-two years earlier for bypass surgery, about the pain he is having now. I barely acknowledge his story, when Howard appears in the doorway in his wheelchair.

It is much later that I recognize how many hours we would have waited for all of this attention had we been at a hospital at home. I recall the night my sister and I sat in the Emergency Room of the same Durham hospital we first approached about Howard's surgery. My friend Susan was in terrible pain from what turned out to be diverticulitis.

We waited for hours, and sometime past midnight, when she still had not been seen by anyone except the police officer standing guard at the door, a young man came in with his head wrapped in a bloody towel. He disappeared behind the double doors. Suddenly the officer announced, "Lock down." We learned the injured man was a gang member, and Security locks down the Emergency Room whenever a gang member is brought in, expecting the rest of his gang to be waiting outside. No one could leave and no one could come in—for hours.

Finally, we got Susan into an examining room, but it was still hours longer before anyone gave her any medical attention. She received a diagnosis, pain medicine, antibiotics, discharge papers, and a hefty bill shortly before 9:30 the next morning, when I finally got to drive her home. I thought then: Next time we'll bring a bottle of ketchup and dump it all over her clothes before we check in.

The neurologist who examines Howard says his eyes are fine now. The ophthalmologist is a beautiful slim blonde woman in pants, high heels, and a sari-type blouse. Her name is Dr. Chandra. She takes Howard into the treatment room (the same room where he was shaved for his first surgery) and looks at his retinas with her light. She tells us everything looks normal now, but dilates his eyes. She will come back later tonight to do a thorough eye exam. It is Friday night. We are told we are not going anywhere, at least until Monday.

"But the Centrum is holding our room," I say.

"Naruna takes care of that," Sister Elizabeth says. "They keep room for you. Now, Mr. Howard gets into bed for heparin. Please."

We learn that the CT scan is normal. Later, Howard is listening to a tribute to Bob Dylan on his Walkman when Dr. Chandra returns to examine Howard's eyes. She is not in a hurry, though I imagine someone is waiting for her at a dinner table somewhere. She finds no damage. She patiently explains about TIAs (transient ischemic attacks) where tiny blood clots break off and begin to travel.

"One may have gotten lodged in your retinal artery," she says.

Dr. Chandra instructs Howard to close his eyes. She leans over him and gently rubs his eyes with her fingers. It is a hypnotic movement. "But the retinal arteries are so tiny," she says, "we know it had to be a tiny clot." Something set it free to move on; thus, the temporary loss of vision, but without permanent damage.

While she massages Howard's eyes, she tells us to call her office next week and make an appointment for a thorough exam, just to be sure. Her office is just around the corner from the Centrum Hotel. How convenient. And if she wears that silky top to work, I'll have no trouble getting Howard to keep the appointment.

"If you feel your vision blurring again," she says to Howard, and looks over at me to make sure I'm watching, "press on your own eyes. Like this."

I write down: Blurred vision = press on eyes.

Howard is a firm believer in massage. It is a regular part of his schedule at home. But never did I suspect that massaging eyes could become part of the routine, or look so intoxicating. I feel my own body relax just watching the circular motion of Dr. Chandra's fingers.

She gives me her business cards and I promise to call next week. Howard gets back into his bed. Sister Elizabeth wheels in another IV pole. Not only are we not moving to a large sunny room with twin beds, but Howard is now flat on his back with a heparin drip in his arm to prevent any clots. I ask how long this will take.

"Until his PT is good," Sister Elizabeth says.

PT stands for prothrombin time, which, rightly or wrongly, I've come to equate with thin blood. "Good" must mean thin enough to prevent the formation of clots. Sister Bindi brings in a pot of steam for Howard. The physical therapist listens to his lungs and says they are fine. In between procedures, I ask Howard what he is seeing.

"I see fine," he says. "I still see a few patterns and lights, but they come and go."

"Still?"

"Yeah. And remember that night Mabel was here?"

I do remember that lovely ICU nurse in greens who first washed Howard's hair.

"All that night I kept seeing her really tiny, lying on her own bed way up high where the TV is."

I just look at Howard.

"I could see her looking down on me from her bed, but I didn't want to disturb her. She was so tiny, like Tinkerbell or something." Howard is slightly amused with telling me this. I am not amused at hearing this now for the first time.

"Today, that thing with your eyes was so scary! Please don't do that again," I say. "Please?"

Howard says nothing. He doesn't even look at me.

Sister Elizabeth returns to adjust the heparin drip.

"Take it out."

I freeze in my place. Sister Elizabeth's eyes are as wide as mine must be.

"Take what out?" she asks Howard.

"The IV," Howard says. He starts to sit up in his bed. "Everything is normal. I am fine. We are going to a hotel. What's it called?" he asks me. "Central? The Center?" He is shouting.

"Howard, please." I recognize a battle I have already lost.

"You must lie down," Sister Elizabeth says. "I cannot take out. You must have heparin for blood."

When she leaves, Howard gets up to go to the bathroom, pulling the IV pole with him.

"Howard, stop! You're bleeding!" Blood drips down his arm, onto his sheets. There are dots of blood all over the floor.

He brings the IV pole back and sits on the edge of the bed. He hangs his head. I can't tell if he is crying or not.

The sisters rush in, clean him up. They try to explain that Howard can go to the bathroom, but they must clamp off the IV first. Otherwise, he is to lie flat in bed. While he is in the bathroom, two sisters change his sheets. No scolding. No drama. Howard resumes his place in bed.

I am so grateful all of this happened here and not at the hotel. What would I have done? Howard could bleed to death before I knew what to do. I remind myself that Naruna suggested we stay close to Escorts. This must be why.

The night is difficult. Howard is belligerent. He finally refuses the heparin drip altogether. I feared he would make a decision that went against the medical advice of these doctors at some point. And here is the first.

Although I want to respect his decision, I am exhausted. I take every opportunity to rest when Howard falls asleep. The IV pole stands beside his bed, the tubing wrapped around and around, hooked only to the full bag of heparin.

Saturday, October 9, 2004

By 6:00 A.M., Sister Reena appears. A new shift of sisters; a new day of energy.

"Good morning. I begin heparin now, and take sample?" she asks. I stop. Hold my breath. Surely the night sisters have told her what happened during the night. Howard refuses.

"But Sister Reena, it is the blood sample that will show if Howard's PT is up to two yet, right?" I ask.

She nods.

"And when it is at two, we can stop the heparin?"

She nods again.

Howard thinks about it. Then he sticks out his arm. Sister Reena takes another blood sample. I do not say a word.

We spend the day working on the thank-you collage for the nurses. Howard stays in bed, and I use one of the alcove counters to lay out pictures and words I have cut from newspapers and magazines. "Meet the pros." "No tomatoes." "Always helping." "We have a new home in India." I hold up the phrases, Howard nods. With a glue stick, I stick them down on posterboard: "The sweet-coated pill." "Chocolate." "Forgive me."

9

PURGATORY

Sunday, October 10, 2004

"I hate this country," Howard says. I try to open my eyes, but everything is moving slowly (except for my bowels). "I'm never coming back here." I say nothing. We are not in discussion mode. We have been in the hospital for over two weeks. Mentally, I practice comforting things to say to Howard. "It's better this way. It's only two days since you began the heparin drip...." Howard doesn't want to hear any of this, I am sure. He feels sentenced, without a satisfactory explanation. The doctors he's seen have told him he is normal.

I feel confused. The system here is clearly one in which Dr. Trehan makes the rules. But Dr. Trehan rarely speaks to us. As smoothly as the rules seem to be carried out, it is disconcerting to not have anyone to talk to, to listen, or to explain the reasons behind actions.

I don't blame Howard for feeling captive, but don't know what to do without creating a complete disaster. I do not want to be out on our own, responsible for Howard's care. I suppose we could pack, get a taxi to the airport. Take the next flight out. Hope we can make it without Howard throwing another clot or starting to bleed. I suppose Howard's cough will be easier on him if he continues the soothing steam treatment as long as it is available. But he must make his own choices, as I will expect to when I am in a similar situation.

There is nothing worse than feeling powerless. I've come here to support him. I've tried to understand as much as possible along the way. Now, I feel in over my head. CNN can just get a different patient to complete their story of the first Americans to come here. I love Howard so much, I am so tired, and I am surprised to find my fists clenched, my jaw tight.

Howard convinces me that we can go. We agree we will return for the official discharge by Dr. Trehan whenever he wants to see us—Monday, if necessary. But we are moving to our hotel. Everyone who comes by hears that we are leaving. We are trying to say good-bye to our friends. They all have similar responses.

"Not today, tomorrow."

"No one goes on Sunday—it is holiday."

"We are not staying in the hospital because Dr. Trehan is off on Sunday," I say. "We only stay in the hospital if we need medical care, and Howard is normal."

I pack our bags again and wheel them out into the room—a statement of sorts. But everything I do takes longer because I am back and forth to the bathroom as if I'd drunk a case of beer. My back aches. Finally, I start my period. Of course. Perfect timing, as always. I'd brought a few tampons with me in preparation of this momentous, albeit inevitable occasion, assuming I could buy an adequate supply once I got here.

I take a tampon to show a sister to ask where I can buy more. The first sister backs up as if it might explode. She shakes her head. I ask another one. She shakes her head and says, "I do not know this."

What? The women in India don't have periods? I ask the head sister. She has never seen a Super Tampax? Obviously, these women have never seen tampons, period. Do they still wear old rags? I give up and decide I will just go to a pharmacy, or as they are called here, to a chemist, and ask. If they don't know about these in a hospital, I can't imagine that anyone will know. This is not a detail Bryan covered with his tips for our travel. Why would he? Who would have thought?

Caught between my own frustration and loyalty to Howard, I ask the next sister who comes by to call for a doctor to come and remove Howard's cannula.

Howard is so thin, so angry. He doesn't do waiting well under the best of circumstances. Finally a doctor shows up. He is short, light-skinned, with eyes that rove naturally; they remind me of Howard's eyes during his "visual disturbance."

"Remove my cannula and this pacemaker," Howard says.

The doctor shakes his head. "Tomorrow we will remove them," he says. "Not on Sunday."

I suppress my urge to scream because Howard screams first. "Take them out. Now!" The doctor looks at me. Howard shouts again, "Take them out, or I'll take them out myself."

I suddenly remember when Naruna said, "Why don't you call me when you have a problem?" So, while Howard argues with the doctor, I pick up the phone and call Naruna. But I get only the message on his cell phone. It is Sunday. He is probably with his family and off duty, as he should be.

Finally, the doctor and sisters who now surround Howard's bed call the neurosurgeon who was consulted when Howard's vision went bonkers. They hand the phone to me.

"The CT scan is normal," I begin. "Howard's vision is normal. The neurologist who consulted said that he was normal...."

"I am the neurologist who examined Howard," the doctor says. His voice is calm. He doesn't say anything about it being Sunday, and I calm down immediately. He explains very clearly in perfect English that what happened to Howard was a mini-stroke.

"Stroke?" I have never heard anyone here use the term "stroke"—not mini or otherwise. He has my attention.

"Fortunately, whatever clot left the valve site, did not lodge anywhere or block anything for longer than the actual time of his visual disturbance. The reason for the heparin is to get his blood to two-and-a-half times as thin as it would be normally."

"And how thin is Howard's blood now?" I ask, forcing myself to picture thin blood and not Howard's stick-thin body.

"He is at 1.86," the doctor says. "They like it at 2.0 to 2.6, but no higher."

"Thin, but not too thin?" I say.

"Yes. To prevent any risk of him having a stroke where the clot may lodge and actually cause some permanent damage."

"Who should have come to explain this to us?" I ask. "No doctor has come since the ophthalmologist who said everything looked normal, see me next week for a field vision test."

"No one explained this?" he asks. "I thought—"

"No," I interrupt. "No one has come to explain anything except that Howard needs heparin and that we can't be discharged from the hospital because it is Sunday. I've never heard the word 'mini-stroke,'" I say. "Now I understand. I will explain this to Howard. Thank you. Dhanyawaad."

I hang up the phone and sit beside Howard on his bed. I try to relay the entire explanation I have just heard, and I can see Howard's body relax as my own has, with resignation. I apologize to the poor doctor who just faced a raging patient (I'm sure not his first) who threatened to leave AMA (against medical advice). "Maph karna," I say to every sister I can find, brown uniform or white. "Maph karna." But these people must learn to communicate better if they expect patients to comply with their orders.

Howard is extra polite to Biji, the sister who takes over on the next shift after Reena leaves. She is thin and dark and shy. She is the sister I heard a doctor become impatient with on our first night here. I had wanted to come to her defense but didn't know how.

Howard stays on heparin except for the time he asks to be clamped off so he can e-mail his son, Alan. When he is finished, I e-mail Dr. Srivastava to explain the nightmare of this weekend. I figure he will hear about it eventually, and it won't be pretty. I hate the thought of him thinking we are being uncooperative, belligerent, or obstinate. He might as well hear it from me.

Later that evening, Howard says he wants to call his good friends Will and Molly. I use the card and our new cell phone that Anuf and Medha from Hospitality got us for when we left the hospital. I wait until we are connected before handing the phone to Howard.

He speaks to Molly in his most ordinary tones, tells her to say hello to the baby, then asks for Will. Howard's face drops. Will is out on a bike ride. Logic would allow for the possibility of his friend not being home to receive a random call from India. But logic is not the primary operating system here. Will's absence is physical and emotional news, and my heart sinks with Howard's.

"Well, just tell him I called, and I'm doing fine. Good talking to you, Molly." I watch as tears fill Howard's eyes. He hands me the phone.

It is really hard to balance offering comfort with allowing a vulnerable person to save face; to not force that person to talk about every unpredictable, random but nonetheless very real emotion that washes over him. I'm sure Howard doesn't want, and maybe even can't, discuss why he feels like crying because Will is out on a bike ride. There is no reason to push the issue. But I don't want to seem indifferent.

As is often the case, he takes care of the awkward moment himself—he swings his legs back up into the bed and opens his book. The phone rings and presents me with a decoy to keep me from being in Howard's face.

It is Dr. Srivastava. He got my e-mail, and immediately begins to explain Howard's TIA.

"From what you said in your e-mail, Howard has the textbook symptoms of a transient ischemic attack; 'transient' in that the clot or particle came and went, leaving no damage and no trace of it." His voice is rhythmic but compassionate. "Should we see any trace or blockage, it is no longer transient. But basically, a TIA is a mini-stroke."

"I understand now," I say. "I wish we'd known this earlier—it could have saved a lot of toes we stepped on, I'm sure."

"Well, you didn't know," he says. "They need to explain things to you."

"It would help."

"Now, about the heparin—there is no magic number," he says. "They only want to reach a degree of safety so Howard doesn't throw another clot, or thrombus, that just might not keep on truckin' without causing damage." Dr. Srivastava explains that this is a common postoperative concern with valve surgery, and it is critical to keep the blood thin enough without being so thin that the patient bleeds spontaneously. They want to safeguard against the risk of stroke that might cause permanent visual impairment or worse.

"I can't thank you enough for calling to talk to me," I say. "I feel like I understand the whole picture now."

Earlier, Dr. Srivastava and I had talked about the need to improve communication among these doctors, which isn't peculiar to Escorts' doctors by any means. I told him about the time, over thirty years ago now, when a doctor told me I had a tumor with a one-in-two-thousand chance of being cancer. Of course, all I heard was the word "cancer" and I couldn't eat or sleep for the weeks that passed before the pathology report (that somehow got lost) was delivered to me.

And all we heard about Howard after his TIA was that everything's normal. Then, instead of helping us understand the importance of staying for the extra days of heparin, we were given excuses like, "You can't leave because it is Sunday," and "We have no discharge on Sunday." I told Howard, I could not picture U.S. insurance companies paying for an extra day because the doctor wasn't there on Sunday to sign discharge orders.

I go to work on the collage for the sisters. I ask Howard to select the placement of photos, and then I glue them down among the words we chose before.

"We should put each of their names on it somewhere," Howard says. "But what real gift can we give them? They have been so patient and steadfast...."

"And so forgiving!" I add.

"How many sisters are there on this floor?" Howard asks. "Let's give each sister some cash for herself. How much? Five hundred rupees each?"

I try to do the math to convert, to guess how many sisters there are who have taken care of Howard. Dozens, that's for sure. I will ask Rita for a list of their names. I will tell her it is for this card, and then we'll count.

"And don't forget the ICU and Recovery sisters," I say. "And what about all the food servers, and the housekeeping guys, and the pest-control guy...."

"And the barber!" Howard says.

"It takes a village to take care of Howard's heart!" I say, spreading my arms out wide.

"No, Hillary," Howard says, "It takes an entire hospital."

My son Thane e-mails from New Zealand where he has finished up his course work for his semester of studying abroad. He is preparing to leave for Australia to camp and snorkel. He is bored, ready to get out of there and see something new, something warm.

I realize my reply is lukewarm compared to how compassionate I usually am when my children seem unhappy. I know it is good to focus on other things, and I surely miss my kids. I do miss them; I miss Susan, Sarina, my sisters, my mom and dad. But I find I have no energy for much besides Howard. Right now, I must focus. I am focused.

Sister Rita calls me from her home to find out how Howard is doing. This off-duty attention is astounding. I cannot think of one sister who has not been competent, pleasant, and totally conscientious about Howard's care. "Sister Rita," I say. "Do you know the names of these trees outside our window?"

"The Neem tree?"

"I don't know," I say. "They have lots of tiny leaves. And the yellow and green birds fly in and out of them."

"Yes," she says. "Neem. It is used for many medicinal purposes from ancient times." Sister Rita speaks very sophisticated English. "The leaves are used for cuts. The bark for fever. And small children chew on the bark or roots for toothaches—you say, toothaches?"

"Yes. Toothaches. I understand." I think for a minute about Howard's hiccups, then ask, "Does any part of this Neem tree fix hearts?"

"Not yet. Maybe someday." Sister Rita laughs. "Oh, and the birds are called 'bee-eaters.'"

"Yes, Bee-eaters. I will write this down. Dhanyawaad, Sister Rita."

By the time the sky darkens to leave a landscape of lights in our window, and I draw the drapes, I feel as though we must be in the homestretch now. Tomorrow, probably everything will change. At least Dr. Trehan will be back. Sumitra brings clean sheets for me and an extra blanket (since Howard wants the air-conditioning so low now), and says good night. I breathe more deeply; at least deep enough to fall asleep before midnight.

I awake to Sister Sumitra and Sister Reena hovered over Howard's bed. I look at the clock. It is 1:00 A.M. Why didn't he call me? Howard is having chest pain.

He describes it to the sisters as traveling across his chest from left to right. "Sometimes in spurts," he says, "sometimes all across here." He traces the line of his incision, which I know is the opposite side from his heart.

Within minutes, two sisters wheel in a portable machine and do a bedside ECG. Dr. Echo comes in to read the report and to examine Howard.

"It is no problem with your heart," Dr. Echo says. "Possibly gastritis or muscular pain." But I am scared, and I am sure Howard is terrified. He has not been in any pain through this entire ordeal; at least none he remembers. Heart surgery and no pain—still an unfathomable concept to me.

When Howard is finally resting again, I walk down the hall to check my e-mail on the computer at the sisters' station. Jackie, our Web designer, sends statistics from the Howard's Heart Web site. On the day the *Times of India* article about Howard traveling to India came out, there were more than 25,000 hits on our Web site. Each day since, the number of hits has declined to anywhere from 1,000 to 10,000 a day. Amazing how quickly word spreads. What I thought would make keeping our families up-to-date on Howard's progress easier on me has turned into global communication.

It's encouraging to read all the e-mails from people we don't even know. The world is cheering Howard on. I send an update for Jackie to post, saying that we plan to be discharged today, and hope to travel to Agra to see the Taj Mahal this week. I must arrange for a driver with Naruna.

I finally return to sleep for a couple of hours before light peeks through the opening between the drapes and divides our room in half.

Monday, October 11, 2004

In the real morning, Howard receives a little heart machine that costs 7,000 something—dollars or rupees. Dr. Trehan has arranged for Howard to get one for free. It's to monitor his heart in case he has any chest pain. A technician trains Howard to use it while I pack the last of our belongings and get the collage ready to present to the sisters on our way out. We fit in two meals before Dr. Trehan calls for us. I am slightly embarrassed to face him after whatever stories he's been told about this weekend's drama. Howard asks me to braid his hair, and chooses to wear jeans, a T-shirt, and tennis shoes. He elects to walk, not ride, down to Dr. Trehan's office.

Dr. Trehan greets us, asks us to sit down. His office is crammed with people who have come to know and love Howard. He has been a big hit, as always, and I look around, amazed at the number of medical professionals who have been a part of Howard's care. Even Dr. Srivastava is here for our parting photo op. He has definitely become my most trusted friend here in Delhi. Dr. Trehan jokes a bit, and then examines Howard. I practice a few of the Hindi words Sumitra and others have taught me, and Dr. Trehan is patient with me.

Howard sits beside Dr. Trehan and asks how he can most appropriately give a financial contribution to the hospital. Dr. Trehan suggests gifting the cost of heart surgery for an Indian child. I have seen the beds come off the elevators with babies so lost in the white sheets that I could barely tell it was not an empty bed. I've heard the children crying, their mothers trailing behind the bed as the sisters move it through the hallways. It is a perfect idea. Howard requires no more options. This is what he will do.

Howard's discharge turns out to be a glorious celebration with photographs and hugs and tears. And we are only moving down the street to the Centrum Hotel. I cannot even imagine how sad the day will be when we leave Delhi. But we have over a week to go, so I dismiss the thought.

We have final orders for discharge—this time for real! Howard and I go downstairs to the Finance Department to pay the final bill, three weeks after our arrival. Dr. Trehan keeps the bill at $6,700, despite a second surgery, all the complications, and the extra days in the hospital for both of us! The Finance Director is noticeably chilly compared to our first meeting. Last Friday night, he'd tried to collect another $5,000 from me, but I refused to pay until I talked with Dr. Trehan. When we are finished and the bill is clear, I ask if we might talk to him in private. He opens the door and we enter the Finance Office. He directs us to a desk with two chairs. Howard explains that he would like to give a gift.

"Could you tell us the approximate cost of heart surgery for a child?" I ask. "In U.S. dollars."

Mr. Finance gets up and runs an adding machine strip that converts rupees to dollars, and hands it to me. Howard and I consider a round number that would be close to this amount, and Howard hands him back his credit card. "Please accept a gift of three thousand U.S. dollars toward a child's heart surgery."

Mr. Finance's face relaxes a bit, and I imagine only now is he sure we are not trying to get away with anything else. He smiles after he has run the credit card through, offers Howard a receipt, and we stand to shake his hand. If I have learned anything by now, it is that we cannot worry about every single person's attitude. We do what we know is right, listen for confirmation, and move on. Howard adds a slight bounce to his step, very slight, but a bounce nonetheless, as he crumples up the receipt, tosses it in a trash can, and we head toward the elevator.

"Howard's heart fund just multiplied and covered two hearts," he says. "Mine and some little Indian child's."

"Like loaves and fishes," I say. Then I remember Howard is Jewish.

We leave through the main entrance, with Naruna and Sanjiv and all the Hospitality folks there to say good-bye. The number of cameras and requests for different combinations of people to stand with Howard for a picture reminds me of a wedding. And it might as well be. We will never have this large a family at any wedding we might have.

The driver delivers us to the Centrum Hotel. We pass many of the places I have seen—the park, the temple or mosque, the bus stand—but I know Howard has seen none of it. He has been in a hospital room for eighteen days, ever since that dark night Sanjiv drove us from the airport. It seems like months ago when I was surprised by cows in the streets. Now, nonchalant, we drive beside them as if cows and cars are sold from the same lot.

10

CUTTING THE CORD

Monday, October 11, 2004

We arrive at the hotel and stand before the desk to check in like real travelers. I ask Howard to sit on a chair that looks out on the street while I hand over passports and sign in for the room they've so graciously held for us over the weekend. Floor fans are on high speed and Howard becomes chilled. He has lost so much weight; there is absolutely no fat left on his body to regulate his body temperature.

The staff are all young men in white dress shirts and ties, nice pants, and polished shoes. They carry our bags, hold the small elevator door for us, open the door to our "room with a view," and turn on the air-conditioning. I open the curtains so Howard can see the bustling street and shops from the love seat. It's like a movie starting up on a blank screen, close-ups of what we've watched from four floors up.

Across the street, a man is sitting on the ground stringing flowers—yellow, red, and white blossoms that look like miniature mums or carnations. The carts and rickshaws that pass under our window feel close enough for us to drop down into them. And once again, Howard is most entertained by the construction workers who ride by on their bicycles with a couple of 2 x 4s under one arm, a short stack of bricks balanced on their heads, or pulling a cart with a few sheets of tin. This window, like our Escorts window, will provide lots of new distractions for Howard.

Once Howard is settled in watching the street scene, I venture out to the chemist across the street to get his prescriptions filled. Actually, no prescriptions are required in India—you just ask for what you want and pay for it. But I've written down the names of the medications Howard is supposed to take on my notepad.

Crossing this busy street is different from crossing the street in front of Escorts, because there is a concrete median, or at least part of one that serves as a midway safety zone. I remember to look the correct way for oncoming traffic, which is to the right, and jump up onto the median before switching to look left. Only then do I realize bicycles and cars turn around in the middle of each side to go the opposite way, at random.

I make it to the pharmacy and tell the chemist I need the blood thinner, which I have learned to call warf 5. There are several other medicines the doctors suggested we get, like a stool softener, a sleeping pill, a pain pill. I also ask for more of the malaria pills I've been taking since I left the U.S. Then, I pull out a wrapped Super Tampax to show him. He looks at me and shakes his head. "Surely women use something!" I say.

He takes it and turns it over in his hands the way I've seen people inspect a cigar, and then sets it down on the glass countertop. He squeezes back behind the other clerk to the very back of the store, which is really more like a covered kiosk, and steps up on a ladder to reach a high, dusty shelf. He brings down a two-and-one-half-inch cube of cellophane-wrapped tampons the shape of OB tampons. They are tampons that come without applicators.

"That's the only kind?" I ask. I despise using these little suppository tampons. He nods. I cannot think of any reasonable alternative, so I accept. I also see a package of sanitary pads in the glass case I'm leaning on. I point to it.

Then the chemist shows me the number and date stamped on the foil pack of the warfarin. Once, someone warned me about always checking the expiration date on medicines I bought in India, to make sure they were in their factory seal. As if I'd know if the seal had been broken. As if I knew the shelf life of warf 5. I nod in approval.

"How much?" he asks.

Is the price up to me? Then I realize he's really asking how many pills I want, not how much I want to pay him. I point to three foil strips, figuring I can always come back for more. He jots down the prices on a scratch pad. In a fairly quick conversion, I figure the total cost for all of Howard's meds and mine. It comes in under four U.S. dollars.

I walk up the street before I cross, looking for water and juice for Howard. He is not to leave the hotel for a few days, just to be safe. (If I could find any takers, I would make bets on the likelihood of my being able to enforce this one!) I wait to go around a rickshaw because a Brahma bull passes first. There are sleeping puppies all over the sidewalk, a man relieving himself in the alley, a woman carrying a huge sack of flour on her head. Everyone stares at me, but why wouldn't they? I am white. I do not carry anything on my head. I do not wear a sari. I hesitate when a bicycle rickshaw cuts in front of me.

I find a stand where I see bottles of water behind the glass, and juice cartons, like the ones that come with tiny straws that I used to pack in my kids' lunch boxes. I get a couple of each, with different pictures of fruit on the front, and I start walking toward our hotel. Navigating the streets is a bit harrowing, often hilarious. Then I see the children, four of them draped all over the sides of the bicycle their father is pedaling. They are giggling, hanging on for dear life, their little bare feet only inches from the spokes. I want to shout a warning. Then I want to weep.

When I walk up the clean white steps of the Centrum Hotel and open the glass doors, the front desk clerk tells me we have a phone call. I ask to take it in my room so I won't be away from Howard any longer. It's a reporter from the *Washington Post*. I agree that we will meet with him tomorrow at 11:00 A.M. for an interview.

Then, Wednesday is the big CNN interview with Dr. Trehan at the hospital, the continuation of my brief interview with them while Howard was in Recovery. Undoubtedly, this interview was arranged around Dr. Trehan's return from the States, and since Howard is walking and talking and feeling pretty normal, we have agreed to return to Escorts to participate.

There is a computer in the lobby of the hotel, so I'm hoping it will be a bit less of an imposition for me to e-mail Jackie regularly. I also realize I must pay my bills online. We've been gone three weeks. Surely some of my bills are due. My parents are stopping by my house to collect mail, so

I ask my mother to send me an e-mail with the amounts owed to my utility companies and credit cards. We've recharged our cell phone, but Howard is still too weak to have much of a conversation. I expect this will improve daily. At least he is resting in a nonhospital bed without guardrails.

Tonight, we will eat our first non-airplane/non-hospital food in three weeks. The hotel manager says he will bring dinner to our room so Howard won't have to go out yet. "We make you hygienic food, as the doctor ordered," he says. I know he is in cahoots with the hospital, or at least with Naruna, and I hope they don't just get Escorts take-out. As good as the food was at Escorts, it will be fun to eat while looking out on a different scene.

"I get overwhelmed when I stop to think of what we've just done," I say to Howard.

"Then don't," he says. He is lying on his bed reading.

I have come to excuse Howard's often curt responses. I tell myself his welcoming, accepting conversations will return with his strength. "Now, we need to think about returning home and how to regulate your energy and breath," I say. "Everyone's going to want to see you. I'm thinking of a sign-up sheet for ten minute visits—one each morning, one each afternoon, maybe one each evening." Howard says nothing.

The phone rings more often than I would've expected, given we know no one in India except the people we just left at Escorts. Naruna calls to warn us of another reporter who wants to talk to us. Some of the sisters call to check on Howard. We grant more interviews with reporters, some over the phone, some I schedule for later in the week.

"Did you notice that newspapers tear the opposite way here?" Howard asks me. He is ripping out an article horizontally which, at home, results in an impossible ragged mess.

I stop and look at him, amazed. This could qualify as small talk. "Yes I did, when I was cutting and tearing out words for your chocolate campaign and for the sisters' thank-you collage." I am encouraged by this detail he has come up with on his own.

We order Chinese food.

I call Sister Rita, the nursing supervisor, to ask how we could give each sister some cash. She checks with her supervisor, and calls me back to say.

"It is not wise," she says. She explains that any money the sisters receive must be put into the general fund, and it won't get spent until most of these sisters have moved on.

We consider slipping them some money to spend on themselves but, finally, we agree that we must think of something else.

In an e-mail, I ask Dr. Srivastava about appropriate gifts. He explains that the equivalent of flowers in the U.S. would be a plate of assorted sweets. I picture baklava and the little pistachio cookies I've eaten at Greek restaurants and Mediterranean delis. I will ask Naruna about stores that sell sweets.

Tuesday, October 12, 2004

John Lancaster from the *Washington Post* calls from the lobby at the scheduled time. With the exception of Suhasini, from CNN, who interviewed me while Howard was in Recovery, this is our first face-to-face interview with a reporter in India. John is a tall, fair American, who is anything but intimidating.

We chat with him in our hotel room, answering his questions about why we chose India and what preconceived notions we might have had about India before we arrived. John is an effective reporter. He is so generous with his personal stories and so obviously interested in us as fellow American visitors to a country he has come to know well, we relax completely. He could ask us anything and we would answer him truthfully and completely. He too was once new here. He tells us about people who come here for dental care at a fraction of the cost of U.S. care.

"You get your teeth fixed and then go to the beach, or see the Taj Mahal. Great way to vacation." He tells us about his children who attend school here. I am impressed with what must be an early global education unmatched by any opportunity in America. I tell him about all the people back home who have helped make it possible for us to be here without any worries, aside from Howard's health.

"We are planning a big Dhanyawaad party for when we get home," I say. "We want to buy traditional Indian dress to wear, and you're invited!"

John mentions that his wife knows where we can buy authentic Indian dress, depending on what we want—silk or cotton. He writes down his wife's name and their home phone number—urges us to call anytime to ask about restaurants, shopping—anything at all.

He is so generous that at one point, I think he may offer to take us shopping. He leaves to keep his next appointment, to interview Dr. Trehan, but asks if he can return in the afternoon with a photographer. Of course he can.

Howard and I agree that after we are finished with John and his photographer, we will venture out to the five-star Crown Plaza Hotel, the fancy hotel I passed on my walk around the hospital, to exchange U.S. dollars and splurge on a real restaurant meal. It will be a luxurious change. Of course, we will take a cab.

Howard and I anticipate John's return, and refrain from snacking even though we get hungrier than we've been in weeks. We are saving our appetites for our first fancy meal at a table set for two. Much, much later that afternoon, John, the reporter from the *Washington Post*, calls from the lobby. His photographer is with him. He apologizes for having been gone longer than he'd expected to be; Dr. Trehan had been most gracious and the interview went very well.

John and his photographer decide to shoot the photos outside in the sun, in front of the hotel. Howard and I pose beneath the palm tree on the front patio. I wonder if the people watching assume we are Hollywood stars. Howard begins to sweat, and looks very tired. But we keep smiling, then say good-bye to our new friends. It is almost 4:00 P.M., and we have not eaten lunch yet.

"Let's go upstairs and get our money and passports," Howard says. "Then we'll go."

"I'm starving," I say. "And I'll bet you must be too."

We hold hands and turn to walk up the white marble stairs, wide as the building itself. Howard takes a step up to the first step, and I feel his full weight against me. I shuffle my feet to get my balance, thinking at first he is being affectionate. "Hey, watch it," I say. "You're going to...." Before I can finish my sentence, Howard stumbles. I try to hold him up with one arm around him, holding his other hand. He is crumbling, weaving left, then right. Howard is in trouble.

I cannot bear his entire weight, slight as it might be since the surgery. I look up and see through the glass doors the desk clerks running toward us. They support Howard up the stairs to the lobby. I'm sure his feet don't even touch the ground. He tries to dismiss this behavior, saying he just got a little dizzy. But his speech is slurred.

"Please, Howard. Just sit down."

"No, I want to go upstairs to our room."

"Howard, please. Sit here and I'll go get our things." I want some time to think. But I don't want to leave him alone. The desk clerk signals that he will help me get Howard up to the room.

Upstairs, Howard sits on the edge of his bed. "Got some water?" he asks.

I sit beside Howard, and open a bottle of water. I offer it to him. "It's probably just the lack of food," I say.

"Yeah. It just got so hot out there, and I felt a little dizzy." All the Ls and Ts are getting jumbled up in his mouth. He reaches for the bottle of water, but it slips through his hand as if I'd greased it with Vaseline.

"Howard, something's wrong." I'm terrified, and trying not to sound critical. I think about the medicine he took this morning with breakfast when he could still walk to the dining room.

"Nothingzwrong," he says in one continuous mouthful. "Letsgoeat." He tries to stand up but falls back onto the sofa.

"Wait a minute," I say. "What about your medicine? Did I give you a whole or a half of that warf, that brown pill?" I realize I didn't cut it in half for him, and I'm sure he didn't do it himself. Howard shrugs his shoulders. He undoubtedly took a whole tablet when he was supposed to have a half. He has come through all this and now I'm going to kill him by not giving him the right dosage of his medicine!

I pick up the phone and call Escorts, fourth floor. Dr. Echo is nearby. I explain what I have done.

"Is his speech slurred?" Dr. Echo asks.

"Yes, and he can't seem to use his right hand," I say. "Is it the warf?"

"That shouldn't make much difference," he says. After a few more questions, he says not to worry. "Call me again if it gets worse, okay? Anytime."

Meanwhile, Howard is trying to stuff another bottle of water into his backpack. He knocks over the books on the closet shelf, clothes hangers fall on the floor. His coordination is completely out of whack. He is giggling, uncontrollably.

I hold my breath.

He insists that we can still make it to the hotel for a meal. I know we must eat, and that actually seems like the quickest solution. Howard makes it to the door without falling. He is like a two-year-old on the loose. I know I can't take my eyes off of him.

Downstairs in the lobby, I ask the desk clerk to call a cab. When it arrives, the clerk helps us inside, and we arrive at the Crown Star Hotel in a matter of minutes. Porters in red uniforms greet us under the overhang at the grand entrance and open the door of the cab. I get out and offer my hand to Howard. He grips the door handle but refuses to take my hand.

One attempt, and it is clear he cannot get up and walk on his own. A porter helps support him on one side, I take the other. We maneuver our way up the steps in a path that most likely resembles tacking on a sailboat. But there is no breeze. I am positive the hotel staff assumes we are drunk. When we get inside, all eyes turn to us. Luckily, we are here before the dinner hour, and it is not a busy time. An attendant approaches us, asks if he can be of service.

"Food," I say. "Where is your dining room?" Howard's body wobbles against mine.

The hotel attendant looks puzzled, understandably so, and points to the far left corner of the lobby.

I want more than the direction. I want help. I feel panic rising in my throat. "It's open isn't it?" I ask.

"Yes," he says. "Enjoy."

I mouth the words "Help me please?" He takes Howard's arm and we half-lead, half-drag him to the dining room and sit at the first table I see. I turn to the maître d'hôtel. "Menus?" I ask. "Do you have menus? Are you still serving?"

"Yes, of course." He talks and moves way too slow for me.

After a blur of trying to order something that Howard feels like eating, is safe to eat, quick to prepare, and will nourish him, Howard is soon trying to spoon shrimp into his mouth. His blue button-down shirt has the pasta's cream sauce and shrimp splattered down the front. I'm tempted to feed him, but I'm also sure he won't stand for it. I offer him a soft dinner roll. Surely he can hold bread in his hand. It drops on the floor and rolls out into the aisle. The waiter comes with another basket of rolls. I try to eat my salad, the first lettuce I've seen in weeks. Then I realize it is probably washed with water they drink here. I am frightened.

"This is good," Howard says, his mouth covered in sauce.

I nod, reeling. This is a surreal world where no one acknowledges the obvious. I have no time to think. I don't even know the questions to ask, let alone the answers. It was a mistake to come here. We should have eaten lunch. But Howard needed food quickly. We need to change money.

Suddenly, Howard announces that he needs to use the bathroom. This, I had not considered. Of course, the restrooms are on the other side of the lobby. I hurry and pay the bill and lead Howard out of the restaurant. Howard is walking with more assurance, so I stand outside the men's restroom in case I hear him fall. I realize I need to go, myself, but decide it is too risky. I'll just wait until we are back at the hotel.

Seeing him emerge from the restroom is like spotting your kindergartner when school lets out. He survived. I grab his arm and we shuffle across the lobby to the Concierge. We exchange a few hundred U.S. dollars into rupees, then head to the main entrance again. At the top of the steps, Howard looks down as if the stairs are a waterslide. The porters open the taxi cab door, but I know we will not make it down without their help. I motion for them to come.

I might be imagining it, but I think they are secretly disgusted and are reluctant to help these drunken Americans. I cannot stop to care. Howard's weight becomes heavier against me. His legs fold under him like a marionette's until he is almost on the ground. I shuffle; try to hold him up. Before we both completely crumble, one of the porters heaves Howard to his feet. I regain my balance. Together we drag him down the steps. We turn him around and lower him into the backseat of the taxi. This time, I am sure Howard's feet never touch the ground.

I tip the porter, and we make it back to our hotel. I consider calling Dr. Echo again, but Howard seems more coherent in our room. I wonder if he just needed food, in the same way that a diabetic's blood sugar can get so out of whack and be so quickly corrected. What I do not wonder about is how ill-equipped I feel to handle this situation.

Wednesday, October 13, 2004

Today is the day of CNN's interview. I call Naruna as soon as I wake up to warn him of Howard's failing motor coordination and speech. "He will need a wheelchair." Naruna tells

me not to worry. He explains that there were so many reporters who wanted interviews with us and with Dr. Trehan, that
he has arranged a press conference. "It will be easier to do it
all at one time," he says. "I'll send a car for you at 10:00."

We manage to get dressed enough for breakfast and
make our way down the elevator to the dining room. Silver
chafing dishes of boiled eggs, toast, and what I call Indian
sopapillas (puffy deep-fried dough) with a spicy potato sauce
are lined up, and at the end, coffee and juice. Howard sits
while I fix his plate in the buffet line—a line which consists
of me alone, assisted by two delightful servers in black pants,
white shirts, and ties.

Howard allows me to tuck in a napkin at the neckline of
his T-shirt. He tries to stab the boiled egg with his fork over
and over again until it rolls off his plate. I catch it in my left
hand before it hits the floor. The coffee is fixed with milk
and sugar as he likes it, but he fights the cup all the way to
his lips. There is more coffee in his saucer and on his plate
than in the cup. I tell myself that caffeine is probably bad for
heart patients anyway.

The servers stand at attention behind their food table, as
if trying to gauge when to intervene. The white tablecloth,
looks like a drop cloth for finger painting by the time we
are done. I leave a hundred rupees for each of the servers,
call out "Kal malenge," and help Howard out of their sight.
Oddly enough, Howard doesn't seem bothered by any of
this. In fact, I don't think he notices any difference in his
motor skills.

About 10:00 A.M. the phone rings. The front desk clerk
says the driver is here from Escorts. We are ushered straight
to Dr. Trehan's office with Howard in a wheelchair. I remind
myself he walked out of here two days ago. I hope someone

notices. I hope someone takes charge of this and says something more than, "Do not worry, Maggi."

We are whisked away to the fourth floor to rest until it's time for the press conference. Naruna's crew shows us to a corner patient room similar to our old room, but even brighter. The sisters are happy to see us, and I am delighted to have backup again. Howard wants to lie down, and is helped from the wheelchair to the bed. Dr. Srivastava calls and is on his way. I definitely want him to be a part of whatever interview we do.

Suhasini and the photographer from CNN arrive at our corner hideaway. I feel even more like celebrities who must hide from the public. Suhasini sets up while Howard naps. We talk about where she wants Howard to sit for this next bit of her story, and she doesn't hesitate: "In the bed is fine."

Howard's responses to her questions about the care at Escorts are brief—so brief, so deliberate, they almost seem canned. But how many ways can you say, "They wanted $200,000 for the surgery at home, so I came to India. I have never been in pain the entire time. The care here is superb. Yes, I would recommend it to other people." Howard, the Howard I know and love, the Howard who did push-ups the morning of surgery, the Howard who stood on the window ledge in our hospital room with electrodes taped to his chest, that Howard is buried beneath some kind of flat translucent seal. Normally he jokes with everyone, but now he seems emotionless, affectless. I pray I haven't lost him. I would drop bread crumbs on the floor if I thought he would follow them back to me.

We eat lunch, or, at least, fool with our trays. Howard is obviously overwhelmed by all the activity. He is even slower to speak than usual, and I become worried about the demands of the upcoming press conference. Quick-fired questions from reporters—Howard unable to keep up? At last, it is time to give it a shot.

We are escorted to the basement, to the same place I attended Dr. K.'s meditation conference. The lobby is once again filled with buffet lunch trays in silver-covered pans. There are cameras and video recorders and more reporters than I have ever seen in one room, except when I've watched a press conference given by Clinton or Bush or Powell. If someone had asked me a month ago if I thought I'd ever be a part of one of these, I would have laughed. I've done things that gained attention before, but not of this size or scope.

We are led into the main auditorium to the front row. Sanjiv removes one of the folding chairs so they can park Howard's wheelchair beside me. There is a long table assembled on the stage covered with white tablecloth, microphones, and water glasses set at each of the three places. Placards printed with Howard's and Dr. Trehan's names are positioned in front of two of the table settings.

I look around for Dr. Srivastava. He will be the third person on stage. He can talk about health care with these newspeople. But I'm worried about Howard being up there alone.

Reporters come to us holding out microphones like peace offerings. Sanjiv and Naruna grant permission for them to approach us. I do most of the talking because Howard cannot. Reporters hand me their cards which I hold like a stack of playing cards. The most extensive interview is with a reporter from Bloomberg. He doesn't act like he is one of a hundred, but talks slowly and clearly, as if he has all the time in the world.

Finally, Dr. Trehan rushes in. He is in blue scrubs, a face mask dangling around his neck. Suddenly, everyone takes a seat and Naruna motions for Howard to come up onto the stage. I watch as Howard stands from his wheelchair and approaches the few steps to the stage. In one of those slow-motion moments, I watch him try to raise his foot over an electrical cable, but instead, he hooks the cord and starts to fall forward. Sanjiv catches him.

"He needs help," I say. No one offers. I get Naruna's attention, and insist, "Help him." Sanjiv and Naruna each take one of Howard's arms and get him up the steps to the stage. Howard is finally seated at the table on the far side of the stage, Dr. Trehan in the center. I consider running up and squatting next to Howard, just in case he starts to crumble. But I am sure Dr. Trehan and the other Escorts folks don't want Howard to appear weak. Naruna motions for me to take the third seat. Me? I look for Dr. Srivastava but do not see him. I walk up on stage, wonder if I should ask Dr. Trehan to switch with me, and finally take the last seat on stage. I am some eight feet away from Howard, so he is on his own. I watch him while Dr. Trehan begins the conference, thanking the reporters for coming, giving some short background information about why we are here, and then opening it up for questions.

Thankfully, much of the media's concern is about health care for the Indian people, and what Dr. Trehan's plans are for more hospitals in other cities in the future. Eventually, it comes to a question for Howard. He has answered the same three questions over and over again, formally and informally. Today is not the day for him to be charming. He is flat. He is pale and I can see sweat forming on his forehead. I could swear he is leaning to one side.

Fuzzy microphones on long poles bob in the audience like additional faces. One reporter asks me a question about the cost at home and what I think should be done about affordable health care. I respond with something clumsy like,

"I don't know how Dr. Trehan keeps costs down at Escorts, but I think I'll reserve that question for after we are back home and Howard is feeling normal again."

The conference is over. We pose for pictures taken of us with Dr. Trehan, and then off we go, back to our hospital room hideout. Howard is not well. He gets into the bed again, and a young doctor comes in to examine him. Afterward, I see the doctor alone in the hallway and describe the events of the last twenty-four hours to him. He says, "Maggi, you must not worry. This is normal recovery." I am too exhausted to be angry.

I feel more alone than I did even when Howard was downstairs and I waited upstairs. He is *not* "normal." He wasn't this bad before Tuesday afternoon when we tried to climb the steps to our hotel lobby. Before yesterday, he could hold bottles of water. He could speak. He could eat his food without a bib. He was walking just fine. The I doubt my own concern.

Once we are in the car, I ask Naruna's hospitality representative who accompanies us if he knows of a place to buy sweets that is not too far away. He suggests Nathu's Sweets, at the Community Center just down the street. I ask him if we can stop there to order sweets for the sisters. I'm surprised by how comfortable I feel asking for this favor, but I anticipate needing help to place an order. He is most agreeable, and tells the driver to stop.

The Community Center is, in fact, very close. It is an open-air shopping mall with wide stone piazzas winding throughout the area. We have to walk around construction workers repairing the walkways and make so many turns I'm sure I will never find this place again. Finally, I see it—a huge brightly lit storefront that reminds me of an ice cream parlor, with red flashing letters across the top—Nathu's Sweets. It is a bakery with restaurant seating.

The Escorts hospitality man speaks in Hindi to the store clerk. He is so patient, trying to understand exactly what I want and then translating it. I order a large sheet cake and ask them to write "Dhanyawaad Fourth Floor" on the top. My escort asks if I want that in English or Hindi, and he writes down both on the order pad for the clerk. I add a platter of assorted sweets, and make hand signals asking for them to heap it up so it is an impressive mountain. None of the individual sweets look appealing to me—many look like sugared gelatin or marzipan—so I ask them to include as many with chocolate as possible. Howard's contribution. My escort gets it all. I was right: I could never have done this without him.

Not until we return to our hotel room does Dr. Srivastava call. He apologizes for not being at the press conference. "I was waiting in Dr. Trehan's office," he said. "They told me he would stop by after his surgery was finished before we went to the press conference. I sat there through the entire press conference thinking he was still operating." Communication breakdown—again!

I tell him how I looked for him, and how surprised I was that he wasn't there. I also tell him about ordering the sweets. "Thanks so much for your suggestion. I will pick it up and deliver it tomorrow," I say. "I wouldn't have known to do that, if you hadn't told me."

We ask the desk clerk about movies for our VCR. Later that afternoon, he brings us *Titanic*. Howard slips in the video and walks toward my bed.

"Where are you going?" I ask.

"I want to lie next to you," he says. This is a first. I did not expect this here or now.

I scoot over when Howard makes some strange animal noise. He lunges toward me, his arms outstretched. But he misses me, misses the bed, and falls between the bed and the wall with a loud thud. He doesn't move.

"Howard?" I'm afraid he is unconscious.

He lifts up his head. "I missed."

"You were aiming for me?" I can't keep from laughing.

"Yeah, and I missed, okay? So can you help me up, or what?"

He is wedged so tightly it takes us several minutes to dislodge him from the crevice.

"Guess I'm not ready to make love with you if I can't even hit the bed," he says.

"It's okay, honey. Let's just watch the movie."

Howard crawls on top of his own bed and lifts up his shirt. I can see the huge bruises from the fall already beginning to decorate his ribs and chest. From our separate beds, Howard and I watch the Titanic go down. Our first blockbuster in Delhi.

Thursday, October 14, 2004

At noon, I take a rickshaw to the Community Center to pick up the sweets. I want to deliver them myself to the hospital, but do not want to go up to the fourth floor. Before I leave the hotel, I call Sanjiv and ask if he can have someone meet me at the entrance who can deliver them to the fourth floor. "And bring a cart, please?" I say.

When I arrive, Sanjiv himself greets me at the guardhouse. He doesn't have a cart, but he has an extra person to help him. He opens the box lid to look at the cake, and his eyes light up like a child's. I see that the words are as I ordered them, "Dhanyawaad Fourth Floor" and also in Hindu characters. Sanjiv urges me to come with him, but I do not want to be the center of attention. I just want the sisters to be surprised and feel appreciated.

"Then will you allow me to take you to lunch?" he says.

"Oh, no thank you," I say. "I must return to Howard." I am standing in the sun after hauling these sweets across the plaza of the Community Center from the shop to the rickshaw. I am dripping wet, and I'm anxious being away from Howard for so long.

I stick a handwritten thank-you note on top of the cake box that says it is from Howard and me, give Sanjiv a hug, and watch them disappear into the hospital with the huge white box with the cake, and the large tray of sweets wrapped and tied with ribbons. I climb back into the rickshaw that awaits me, feeling considerably less elegant than Cinderella in her pumpkin coach.

At 4:30, we go by cab to see the eye doctor Howard has been referred to for his complete exam. There is no residual damage from his TIA. We return to the hotel room with a hefty packet of charts and diagrams of Howard's eyes to deliver to Dr. Engel back home.

Dr. Chandra, the beautiful ophthalmologist who examined Howard in the hospital, calls to see how the examination went. After we discuss Howard, I ask her to recommend a place to eat that is nearby.

"Howard wants pizza," I say. What I don't say is how hopeful I am that he can get a piece of pizza to his mouth without dropping it in his lap.

"Ego is a good place in the Community Center," she says. "Do you know where that is? It is just around the corner from you."

"Is it the same place where Nathu's Sweets is?" I ask. "I was just there today."

"Yes. Just on the other side of the plaza. Ego is very good."

Howard and I make an outing of it. The way I think about going out with Howard is a lot like the way I thought about taking my boys anywhere when they were toddlers—preparing for almost any unforeseen event, scheduling around meals and naptime, allowing enough time to get home before everyone crashed. With Howard, it is even more unpredictable, because he fluctuates from being absolutely fine to being noticeably impaired. "Impaired" seems so permanent, and I pray that this is not, but Howard definitely has lost some function, both physically and mentally.

He exhibits a distinct loss of strength and motor function on his right side, which means he often drags his right foot, cannot open the water bottle, turn the door key, or carry much of anything without dropping it. Neither his speech nor his memory is up to par, but in this setting, it is easy to make allowances for both.

But when I picture him back on the job, the deficit seems obvious. His loss of function is frightening. As a builder and cabinetmaker, precision and speed are critical. Howard is anything but precise and quick now. I try to hold on to images of him measuring and ripping 1 x 6s, and of him climbing ladders, and cutting and laying tile quickly before the adhesive dries.

I flag down an auto-rickshaw and negotiate the price for the driver to take us to the Community Center (based on what the desk clerk tells me it should cost). We get out in the middle of the street, and make our way slowly past the women and children begging in our path. They make the homeless in New York City look clean and healthy. I remember the Light Child from the park, and wonder if he sleeps there, or here. I wonder which of these women could be his mother.

We find Ego easily and are greeted by very friendly young men. There is a bar area with a sound system, beer advertisements, and a TV turned to the evening news, then an adjacent restaurant area that opens to a kitchen with brick ovens.

"Do you want to start here at the bar?" I ask Howard. I am surprised by my question, it seems so normal.

"Sure."

I make sure we can sit at the bar and move to a table for dinner later. Then I order a beer. A real beer! We aren't sure whether Howard should drink alcohol, so he orders juice. Funny how this question has not come up before. Funny what you get used to, I think.

Our drinks come and the waiters seem amused watching us. Howard tastes my beer. Suddenly one of the waiters points to the TV. We turn and see Howard on the screen. The news is on.

"Hey," he says, "That's me."

The waiters come closer and in easy-to-understand English, ask us why we are here. We are comfortable talking with them.

Howard picks up a slice of pizza, and eats it, no problem. By the time we finish off the pesto pizza that becomes one of our favorite non-Indian meals, the Ego staff have become our friends. They open the door for us to leave, and take Howard's arm to help him down into the now-dark plaza.

We walk through the Community Center to the street. It is much more crowded than when we arrived, and the tangle of rickshaws and cabs seems impenetrable. I watch for an empty rickshaw to carry us back to the hotel.

Howard says, "Let's walk back."

But I know he is tired and doesn't really know how far it is. What I do know is it is much farther than he has walked since his surgery. I decide the goal is to make it across this intersection through traffic busier than we've ever seen it, probably because of the late hour—people on foot, rickshaws going every which way, dogs, beggars, taxicabs and bicycles. On the other side, we will stop and make a plan. I have a firm grip on Howard's arm. A car turns the corner in front of us. A woman waves to us through the back window, and I recognize her. "Howard, look. It's one of your dietitians!"

He is too slow to turn around, and the car is gone. We keep moving with the flow of this river, the other side of the street in sight. I am leading Howard when I feel a hand on my shoulder. I turn to see her, the young woman who took Howard's meal order so many times.

"Come," she says. "We take you to your hotel."

"Oh, it is not on your way. Our hotel is that way," I say, pointing the opposite way their car turned.

"We take you."

We make it to where her boyfriend or husband has stopped the car. There is really no pulling over in Delhi; you either stop or go. We climb in the backseat and I thank the man.

"You are so kind," I say.

He smiles. "Where is your hotel?"

Howard's dietitian turns around to face us. "Is it the Centrum?"

"Yes. The Centrum," I say, surprised that she knows this.

"Just this way," she tells the man.

"Thank you so much," I say.

It is the man who says, "Please do not thank us. We are happy to take you. There is no need to thank us."

Back in our room again, I am so grateful for these kind people. I could have just gotten us into big trouble, trying to walk farther than Howard could walk, or standing there trying to get a rickshaw until he collapsed. I have to be more careful. It is not so easy at night; it is not so easy with Howard.

Friday, October 15, 2004

Dr. Trehan summons us to his office for Howard's final checkup and to be officially discharged from his care. A driver from Escorts comes for us at 10:00 A.M. There, in Dr. Trehan's office, a news broadcast of Howard and me at the press conference from two days ago is on a portable TV screen. I'm the only one who finds the caption under my picture amusing: "Mrs. Staab" it says, as I ramble on about the difference in cost between the U.S. hospital and Escorts.

I remember that everyone assumes we're married, but until this moment, I have never signed anything with my last name as Staab, nor have I seen it in print. I've gone by a few different surnames in my lifetime, but never Howard's.

The chief's office is all abuzz—staff, Naruna, telephones ringing, a cameraman, and the dozen or so monitors of patients' vital signs. Howard's condition is, of course, the reason we are here. Dr. Trehan examines Howard. He assures us that Howard is regaining strength and energy every day, orders a weekend of rest, and says we may then visit the Taj Mahal.

Naruna will make arrangements for us to journey to Agra to visit the Taj Mahal on Monday. Finally, we will begin acting like tourists and see India, at least one building outside of Delhi, and a gorgeous wonder of the world, at that. Then we will return to the States next week. But I have something to say, and it is going to take some maneuvering to get a word in. I play back again Dr. Engel's charge: "Maggi, you are going to have to be assertive."

Dr. Trehan turns his head for a moment, and I go for it. "Dr. Trehan, I must tell you something before we go."

He nods in my direction while one of his staff hands him a phone. He carries on a conversation about flying somewhere, then switches to a chair near Howard, edges forward. I interrupt again.

"Dr. Trehan, I really must tell you what happened."

"Oh, yes. Of course."

I feel an unsettling hush come over the room, and I suddenly feel responsible to "make this good," to make it worth quieting down the entire room and stealing so many minutes of Dr. Trehan's packed schedule.

"We were walking through the Community Center last night after eating at Ego, Dr. Chandra's suggestion."

"Yes, I know Ego," Dr. Trehan says. "Good pizza." I try to imagine him eating pizza, having a beer with us.

"I was trying to find an empty rickshaw to carry us back to the hotel," I continue. "Howard was determined to walk, but I knew he was very tired. Traffic was busier than I've ever seen it, but we had not been out at night before." I try to determine if Dr. Trehan is really listening or if his mind is on any one of a million other things. "I had a hold of Howard's arm as we inched our way into the street when a car turned the corner. A woman waved to us out the back window."

Dr. Trehan's gaze is fixed on me now.

"I said, 'Howard, look. It's one of your dietitians!' But we had to keep moving, trying to cross over so we could stop and think about what to do next. I was leading Howard through the traffic and felt a hand on my shoulder. I turned to see her, the young woman who stood before Howard so many times before a meal asking, 'Indian or Continental?' 'Come,' she said to us. I tried to steer Howard around to follow her to her car where her boyfriend had pulled over to wait for us. 'We will take you to your hotel,' she said."

Dr. Trehan looks behind him at his staff. "Who was it?" he asks. Everyone shrugs their shoulders.

I continue. "They drove us home, Dr. Trehan. And it wasn't easy. It wasn't on their way, and they had to stop in all of that traffic, find a spot to stop and wait, and come and find us to lead us back to their car. They were on a date, and she stopped to help us!"

"What is her name?" he asks me.

"I don't know," I say. "I wish I did. She just always came to ask Howard what he wanted for his next meal."

"Who is this woman?" Dr. Trehan asks his assistants. His eyes have a new light in them, like a father proud of his child's behavior.

If I said she is a beautiful Indian woman with long dark hair, that will hardly help identify this Good Samaritan, but it is all I know. Then I remember the flat tooled leather shoes she wore in the hospital ... that won't help either.

"We'll find out," Dr. Trehan promises.

I'm afraid he will cut me off here, so I force my way onward. "And we have received several calls from the sisters on their days off—from their homes! Sister Deepti called one morning just to make sure I had eaten breakfast. Sister Rita called on Sunday. The nursing supervisor called us at the hotel to ask how Howard was. Your staff has been so attentive. I just want you to know."

Dr. Trehan visibly relaxes against the back of his chair, a posture so casual for him, we might have just as easily been discussing a movie we'd both just seen.

I know I have his real attention now. "I remember the story you told at the press conference about Ch.... I can't remember the name, about the woman who saved the tree."

Dr. Trehan nods with a slight grin on his face. "Chipko," he says. "In Hindi 'chipko' means to cling. The protesters trying to save the forest threw their arms around the tree trunks designated to be cut and refused to move."

"Yes," I say, "Chipko. That's it!" For this moment, he is all mine. "You said you tell all your employees, 'Put your arms around your patients and protect them. Do not let them go.' I think it works."

I picture the EPA's bumper sticker "Hug a tree." I imagine an Escorts Heart Institute sticker that says, "Hug a Patient" or "It is 7 o'clock. Do you know where your patient is?"

"Thank you for telling me," Dr. Trehan says, answering another phone call. When he lifts the receiver into the air for someone to take it away, he says, "Have you seen the movie *Bride and Prejudice*?"

When the Escorts driver pulls up in front of our hotel to drop us off, our new friend Raj is also getting out of his little white car. With him is Mahendra, the friend from Jodhpur who called me at Escorts to check on Howard and two friends. Raj and Mahendra visit with us in the lobby. One of the hotel clerks brings water for all of us. Mahendra presents us with a box of sweets, and I'm proud that I already know what sweets are. Raj pulls out a bag of fruit.

"You come to my city," Mahendra says.

"We would like to," Howard says.

"Tomorrow I go back to my home," Mahendra says. "You come Monday. Fine?"

Monday? He offers to fly us to Jodhpur to tour his furniture factory. Jodhpur, the Blue City. Hopefully, we can still drive to Agra to see the Taj Mahal on Thursday, and then back to Delhi to rest for our flight to the U.S., which leaves on Friday at midnight. We have seen so little of this enormous subcontinent, and we want so desperately to see more, that we accept his offer. When they leave, Howard and I talk about the trips. He is more excited about seeing the furniture factory than he has been about anything since his surgery. I call Naruna and tell him our change of plans. He will try to arrange the trip to Agra for Thursday.

Over the weekend, Howard and I sit on our love seat, and I lay out the Scrabble tiles on the glass coffee table.

"Let's turn these over," I say.

Howard looks at me as if I've asked him to do twenty push-ups. "All of them?"

I consider this. "I know. Let's turn them facing up until we can spell the word 'heart,'" I say.

"I'm sick of my heart."

"Too bad," I say. "Start turning."

As I'd predicted to myself, Howard fumbles with more tiles than he actually turns over. Several fall on the floor.

I remember helping my aunt pick up coins after her stroke. It was her right side, too. I turn tiles over slowly, wondering if the right side is more often affected by strokes than the left. "Next time, we'll try turning over coins," I say.

We watch the movie *Gandhi* in spurts, with naps in between. Mahendra calls on Sunday and tells me that for Monday, all flights from Delhi to Jodhpur are full, but there are seats for Tuesday. Tuesday it is: our first test flight to see how well Howard's heart flies.

THE TRUE INDIA

Saturday, October 16, 2004

Howard and I pick Lodi Gardens as the one tourist attraction we should see, in Delhi, if no other. John Lancaster, the *Washington Post* reporter, actually mentioned it as his favorite—a peaceful place to walk and just relax. He said there was a restaurant nearby where we could eat when we got tired. I try to hire a cab, but none seem available. Howard suggests we can make it in an auto-rickshaw.

"It isn't far. John said maybe fifteen or twenty minutes," Howard says. "Just up by where the eye doctor was."

This seems a little far to me, all that jarring and bumping along. I'm not sure it's such a great idea for Howard to ride very long like that. Plus, since it's open, it will be extremely hot without any way to escape the fumes of the constant traffic. But I find an autorickshaw waiting in the street, the driver has no passengers. "Lodi Gardens," I say.

He nods and smiles. "Lodi Garden." Everyone knows where Lodi Gardens is. It is on every tourist map, in every book I've read. We climb in.

Thirty minutes later, I ask the driver if we are close. He nods. Forty-five minutes later, I know something is wrong. I don't know if I should be angry or scared. John definitely said it was "close." This ride is not doing Howard's heart any good, and we are stuck in a traffic jam on the top of an overpass. We've passed Central Market, which I remember on the map to be way beyond Lodi Gardens.

The rickshaw driver pulls into a gas station. "Wait here," he says motioning for us to get out of the rickshaw. Without understanding, we get out because there are other passengers getting out of and back into other cabs and rickshaws. We wait in the relentless sun while the driver waits in his own queue to get gas. Apparently, no passengers may stay in the car while the driver refuels. When he is finally done, we get back in, and I ask again how much farther.

"Not far." He drives another fifteen minutes and pulls over to a sprawling factory, or industrial plant. He holds out his hand and says, "Passports?"

"What?" I'm becoming impatient with this man's surprises. In the banter of broken miscommunication, the best I can discern is that he thinks we have an appointment at whatever place this is. For him to wait for us, he wants our passports. I have no intention of giving him the passports, even if we had them with us—which we don't—and no intention of riding with this guy on the return trip.

I finally figure out he has driven us three or four times as far as from where Lodi Gardens is to a place called Lodi-

Something-Else-Very-Similar, for diplomats or buyers or something related to the government.

"I said Lodi Gardens!" My voice is in ascension mode. "I said it over and over again. You said it back to me. Lodi Gardens!" I swear our driver is holding back a smile as he faces forward again. "This is not funny!" I point to Howard even though the driver is not looking at me. "He is not supposed to be riding this far, breathing all these fumes. He just had heart surgery. We wanted to take a relaxing walk!"

Howard just sits there. The driver turns around and starts pleading with Howard. Of course, we do not understand much, except he thought this is where I said we wanted to go.

He drives us back to Lodi Gardens, another thirty minutes of bumping and thick, choking fumes. When he finally pulls into an entrance to the Gardens, it is obviously the right place. But by now, my fists are clenched tightly around the metal post, and we have no water left in our bottles. I am furious. The driver stops.

We get out, and I pay him what we agreed on.

He starts screaming at me to pay him much more for the long ride. At first I can't close my mouth or make any words come out of it. Then they come. It isn't pretty. This crook takes us where we do not want to go, for a ride Howard should never have been subjected to, and he wants me to pay extra, beyond what he told me back at the hotel? I don't think so.

We walk away from the rickshaw. I feel horrible about not only the ride, but the driver, the Gardens, and the prognosis for the day, given the length of time between Howard's naps and need for food.

Suddenly, Howard lets go of my hand and turns around.

"Where are you going?" I ask him.

He says nothing. I watch in complete disbelief as Howard fishes out a crumbled bill from his pocket and gives it to the driver. The driver smiles, and drives off. Howard turns back to me.

"So now you're in charge?" I say.

"He misunderstood."

"He did not misunderstand. He repeated Lodi Gardens to me. He gave me the price for Lodi Gardens, not that government place. I paid him what he told me it would be. It was easier to get more of our money than to look for a new trick."

"Maybe." Howard continues to walk into the Gardens. "But he needs the money."

"Since when do we support people who take advantage of us?" I start to walk after him. "And since when do you undermine what I do?"

Howard walks on ahead of me. I follow. I figure this is the first day he has felt in control of anything in a long time. But I know we normally agree on generously tipping those who do their job well, and do not condone dishonesty.

Howard wanders down the path, climbs up to examine old buildings. I follow. I am frustrated and disappointed in our outing and in what I now see is the beginning of a new balancing act with Howard.

"I'm hungry."

"Of course you're hungry," I say. "We've been traveling all day. John said there was a restaurant at the end of the Gardens, remember?"

"I don't see one," Howard says. "Let's get a cab."

"To where?"

"To a restaurant."

Howard leaves me standing there, and crosses the street outside the Gardens. I watch in stubborn disbelief, as he approaches a gaggle of taxis, the cabbies outside polishing their hoods and windows. Where is he going to say he wants to go? To a restaurant? Neither of us knows the name of any restaurant except at the Community Center.

Howard talks with one man, then motions for me to come over to that side of the street. I obey against my better judgment. I have no idea where to tell him to take us. I am positive Howard has even less of an idea.

"Escorts Hospital," Howard says.

The cabbie nods. I want to cry. I want to scream. I want to go home. There is no restaurant near Escorts that we should eat in. There are only the food vendors with the little boys dunking dirty tin platters into trash buckets of water before reusing them to serve more food. Howard is in control mode, but he has no idea what he's doing. How could he? I climb in the backseat with Howard, concentrating on not losing it.

In twenty minutes, the cab pulls up to the corner of the park and Escorts. Somehow, the sign of the hand and red heart is more comforting now than it was when Howard was in surgery. I am seething but silent, waiting to see what Howard has in mind.

"Go on down there," he says, pointing to the direction of the construction I walked through on my search for the Lotus Inn.

"Howard, there are no restaurants down there. I've walked it. It's all under construction."

"There have to be restaurants down here somewhere," he says.

I know how desperately he wants to be right. But I know the road ahead ends up in rubble of concrete and sand under the overpass.

"We'll get out here," Howard says. The driver stops in the middle of the street. Howard pays the cabbie. I thought having us both carry money would be an empowering equalizer for Howard. I consider how different this would be now if only I had kept money in my fanny pack. We both climb out. The taxi drives off. We stand in the street in clouds of dust with construction workers carrying bricks on their heads.

"Howard, please. Let's go into Escorts. We can eat in the Coffee Shop or they have a cafeteria, I'm sure. All these patients' families must eat somewhere."

We start to walk back toward the intersection.

"I'm going this way," Howard says. He takes off across the street in the direction I walked when I was looking for markers and paper and the wine shop. It is where I found the photocopy store and where the boys stitch comforters on the ground. There are food vendors but no restaurants for tourists.

"Howard, please." Begging is never pretty, but I am begging. "It is air-conditioned in Escorts. Let's at least sit down, get a bottle of water, and ask someone."

Howard leans forward as he leaves me. My feet seem to sink into the ground where I stand. I will not follow him. Not this time. "I will be in Escorts lobby," I call after him. Howard disappears into the crowd. I feel tears running down my dusty face. I have never felt so lost, so helpless, and so guilty, all at once. And here I stand right outside the fence of the place we lived for three weeks.

Eventually, I go inside. I need to use the bathroom if nothing else. Sanjiv and Medha and Anuf are all standing around the Information Desk in the lobby, the lobby where I first met Raj. I see their smiles, and then they all rush over to me. I must look like a lost orphan from the streets with the same streaked face as the Light Child.

"Where is Mr. Howard?" they all ask.

"He is walking. He left me." I am crying, the way I cried the day I had to sign for Howard's second surgery. I don't want to do this. I don't want to live through this next day.

"Come," Sanjiv says. "We will go in the car to find him."

Find him? In Delhi? I follow Sanjiv because I do not know how to argue this one. Sanjiv asks me where I last saw him, what he was looking for, and then, why did I leave him.

"You should not leave him," Sanjiv says to me. "It is not good." Sanjiv is the first person to acknowledge that Howard might need me for anything; a bittersweet message.

"But he wouldn't listen," I say. "He needs water and food."

"Yes, he should not walk alone. You should not leave him."

Sanjiv gets the Escorts car. He tells the driver to stop everywhere he knows there is a restaurant. Each time, he gets out and goes inside. I wait in the car, watching for Howard in the street. We drive to the back side of the Community Center. Sanjiv tells me to come, tells the driver to wait. We race from restaurant to restaurant, new ones and Ego and even Nathu's Sweets where we bought the sweets for the fourth-floor sisters. It is midafternoon and most places are empty. Sanjiv speaks to each host in Hindi; I assume he is asking if they have seen an American with long brown hair.

Finally, Sanjiv turns to me. "There is no other restaurant. We go back to your hotel."

The guys at the Centrum Hotel look quizzically at me but say nothing. It is obvious I have been crying. I am without Howard. This is not rocket science.

"Has Mr. Howard been here?" I ask at the desk.

"No. He leaves with you this morning."

I begin to explain but the guilt is exhausting.

I say to Sanjiv "I will wait in our room at the hotel. Please call me if you hear from him or see him."

Sanjiv hugs me and says to call if Howard comes. *If Howard comes.* What have I done?

He leaves in the Escorts car. I pull the desk chair over to the big window in our room. The vigil begins. I try to imagine Howard walking over the garbage in the street, stumbling, maybe having another mini-stroke. An idle mind is dangerously imaginative. There is a scripture in the Bible that says something about an idle mind; of course I can't remember it.

I stare at the street until the sky turns a shade or two darker. Howard is wandering at night. I think of what Sarina would say if she were here: Imagine Howard walking in the door. Imagine him healthy and smiling, leaning down to hug me. I try to picture him pulling up in a cab and looking up to wave at me in the window.

Hours later, Sanjiv calls to ask if I have heard from him. I think of Alan and my parents and all of Howard's friends. It would have been easier to explain a failed surgery than how I lost Howard in Delhi. The later it gets, the more I wish I could hand someone a switch just to beat me till I lose consciousness.

Cabs and private cars pull up to the front of the hotel. With each one, I imagine Howard in the backseat, opening the door and getting out. Finally a rickshaw pulls up and a man gets out. It is Howard. He pays the driver and walks up the steps without help. I am at once relieved, furious, and rebellious, and desperate to not display any of these raging feelings. What I want more than anything is to escape out the back door, let Howard come home to an empty room, and wonder where I am. But there is no door, except the one Howard walks through.

"Hello," he says. He is deliberately quiet.

None of the words I think to say will sound as they need to sound. I cannot make myself speak beyond, "Hello."

"I had a nice seafood dinner," he says.

Sunday, October 17, 2004

Howard is silent. We go to breakfast together with minimal conversation. Howard actually doesn't seem angry, he seems a little blue. He says he wants to read. I am restless. I certainly do not want a repeat of yesterday. So, I decide to go to Central Market, the busy chaotic market I've read so much about. I hire an auto-rickshaw and leave Howard reading his book.

I look at earrings, shoes; see a purple jacket I recognize from the Cold Mountain catalog. I wander, and so does my mind. This is not how I wanted to experience India. I'd imagined Howard and I would pick out souvenirs to take back to Mom and Dad, to our children, our friends, to Jim for mowing the lawn, to Wayne for supervising Howard's crew, to Susan for keeping my cats, to Norman for checking on Howard's kittens. I was eager to barter with the vendors. I imagined we would get tired and stop for a meal and a beer and laugh about how well we had done.

Instead, I am hot, hungry, thirsty, and not interested in buying anything, afraid to eat or drink anything being sold at the stands. At least I've seen Central Market; I compare it to El Rastro, the flea market in Madrid. I buy a new wallet because mine has broken. I decide to leave and wind my way through the tiny alleys between shacks, trying to find my way out of the market to a main street.

The last stall I come to has a pair of shoes like those Howard's dietitian wore—flat pumps of soft tan leather with hand stitching on the toe. I want dark leather, not light. I ask the owner if he has the shoe in a darker color. He says, "No problem. I make dark." He takes both shoes and drops them into a number ten size can of dark liquid sitting in the corner. It is oily and potent, and I realize it must be dye. He leaves the shoes soaking while I pay, 700 rupees (almost $14). With tongs, he takes them out, wraps them in newspaper, sets them in a plastic bag, and hands them to me, grinning and proud. "See?" he says. "Magic. Now, you have dark."

I accept this smelly parcel, and hold it away from me as I walk toward the noise of traffic. I do not know how I am going to stand the overpowering smell, like turpentine or gasoline. And I am so thirsty. I begin to feel queasy. I spot a stand with neat rows of bottled water. I ask the vendor how much and ask to see the seal. He points to it, takes my money, and I walk away to find an empty rickshaw. I just want to go home. I climb in the first rickshaw I see, explain again where I need to go. "Toward Escorts Hospital," I say. "The Centrum Hotel," though I have learned that no one knows where our hotel is.

I settle in for the ride, put the toxic shoes on the floor, and step on the bag so it won't go flying out the door. Finally, I can have a drink of water. I twist off the top, but it is too easy. I've bought a refilled bottle of water even after Bryan warned me, even after I asked to see the seal. Clever. Somehow, clever doesn't impress me at this moment. I've been had. Two days in a row. And I still have Howard to reckon with.

The rickshaw driver actually takes a path as direct as I can imagine to the recognizable street in front of the Centrum. I pay him what we agreed on and hand him the undrinkable bottle of water. A tip of sorts. Howard will be proud.

Howard is asleep when I open the door to our room, but opens his eyes when I shut it. He sits up. His book is still opened on the bed.

"How was your book?" I ask.

"I get tired reading," he says. "But it's okay. How was your day?"

I can only hope that the edge between us is softening more than it seems to be. "Okay. Central Market is one crazy place. I doubt you would have enjoyed it," I say. "Have you eaten?"

"I had some of that juice you bought."

We order an omelet from the room service menu and split it. We sit on the love seat with the drapes open, watching the traffic below. And while we eat, we talk about what else we want to do in Delhi before we leave. We decide that tomorrow, I will call John-the-reporter's wife to ask where we should shop for Indian clothes.

"Think we should get matching outfits?" I ask.

"Sure," he says.

We really don't resolve anything. Yesterday's quarrel dissipates quietly, more out of necessity than anything else.

Monday, October 18, 2004

After breakfast, we arrange with the front desk to have Rajul, the hotel's driver, take us to Fab India to buy our clothes for the Dhanyawaad Party we will have when we get home. He drives us to a small shopping plaza and parks. He will wait—I do not know what he will do while he waits in this heat, but he will wait. We have him booked for the required minimum of four hours. He is ours.

Howard and I see that Fab India has a silk store on one side of the street and a cotton store on the opposite side of the street. We choose the cotton side, which happens to be under construction. So instead of walking in at street level, I must lead Howard down steps covered with plywood into a basement room. The walls are made of open shelves marked with the names of the pieces of clothing: *kurta* (tunic), *mini-kurta* (short shirt), *pajama* (drawstring pants).

I've written down the names of what I need, but don't see the dupatta—the long scarf that wraps loosely around the neck. The place is crowded with shoppers pulling out items, trying them on, rummaging through open boxes on the floor, looking in mirrors. Fortunately, I find a wooden box for Howard to sit on. I hurry, but get confused as to how to correctly put an outfit together. So I ask for help.

A woman explains that most often women will choose the mini-kurta, then pajama pants to either match or contrast, and then pick a dupatta to tie them together. After only a few tries, I choose an orange and purple mini-kurta with short sleeves. I reject wide-legged pajamas, and opt for bright orange cotton pants that could fit both of us inside the waist, but taper down and gather tightly around my ankles. Howard approves.

Now for the dupatta. Some are folded on hangers and look like wide pants. Others are tossed like seconds into bins. Howard picks up a bright orange one with the same purple stripe, and tries to wrap it around my neck. A couple of women pass and say, "Beautiful combination." Done.

I lead Howard over to the men's side where there is much less to choose from. He looks at me and says, "Let's go eat something. I can't do this now."

We must stand in line to check out of the basement with the merchandise, and then go up the steep stairs to stand in line to pay. But soon enough we are out on the walkway with sunlight and air. Howard chooses a place called Bread and More where we get a roll and coffee. Afterward, Howard is rejuvenated and agrees to climb back down into the Fab India basement for his party clothes. He picks an orange striped long-sleeved shirt and bright blue pants and walks over to the full-length mirror to see how he looks.

"Those are the colors you just painted your house!" I say.

"I must like them, really truly, deep down inside." Howard pulls off the shirt.

"Know what?" I ask. "Your bathtub is also orange and blue!"

Howard thinks for a minute. "Didn't even remember that," he says, "and I painted that tub eight years ago."

Carrying our new outfits, we find Rajul and tell him to take us to Khan Market. Howard is doing so well, I can't decide if I should cut this outing short to prevent disaster or go along with it, since we never know when he'll have another "spell." He insists we will keep going.

Howard buys a finely carved elephant for Alan who, at sixteen, has already demonstrated fine woodworking skills. The elephant is carved so deep, we can see inside her belly where there is another even smaller elephant. A ship-in-the-bottle trick; this time made of rich and delicate wood.

I find a tiny store of trinkets and am captivated by the shopkeeper's stories of myths and good luck symbols. I listen and remain undecided about my purchases long enough that Howard announces he is leaving to find a bathroom. I hesitate to let him venture out alone, but he is behaving normally, so I don't argue.

Finally, I choose a dancing elephant, a frog holding a coin in its mouth, and a string of coins to hang by the door to bring wealth. Howard isn't back yet. I pay the owner and step outside. I have no idea where Howard went.

I look for Rajul. He is standing by his cab in the sun. When I turn back to the shops, Howard is coming out of a bookshop.

"There you are," I say. I don't want to sound like a mother who just found her runaway toddler. But that is exactly how I feel.

"Worried?" he asks.

"No, of course not."

"I just climbed three flights of stairs to use the bathroom," he says. "We should go in there. It's an interesting store."

"Some other time. I'm tired though. Ready to go?" I can't believe I am the one suggesting we call it quits.

"Yeah, I'm ready," Howard says.

We climb into our cab with bags of our purchases, and tell Rajul we are ready to go back home to the Centrum. At this moment, we could have been in Los Angeles or Chicago, shopping for souvenirs, returning to our hotel. I am struck by how few of these moments we've had here. "Getting hungry?" I ask.

"Sure. Let's drop these off at the hotel and have Rajul just take us on to the Community Center," Howard says.

"Okay. Do you know what you want to eat?"

"Indian," Howard says. "That place we keep passing called 'Dawar' something, across from the Internet place."

It feels so odd to have Howard directing the evening without things getting out of hand. He suddenly seems so capable, so much like the man who has stolen my heart. So deliciously odd. It is so sweet I want to roll this moment around in my mouth without sucking on it, so it lasts a long, long time.

Tuesday, October 19, 2004

The manager at the hotel agrees to keep our room for us since we will be gone to Jodhpur for just one night. We take only the essentials we need to travel, leave the rest behind. I leave a bag of dirty laundry which, when we return, will reappear miraculously clean and folded. We've heard that people called *dhobi wallahs* (laundry servants) come and collect dirty laundry, and then go to the river to wash the clothes before returning them to the hotels to distribute them to their owners. Apparently, it's true.

We take a cab to the airport after breakfast. Nothing looks even slightly familiar, and I assume we are leaving from a different airport than where we arrived in Delhi. It makes sense, since this flight to Jodhpur is a domestic flight and ours was an international flight.

Mahendra and another man pick us up in Jodhpur and drive us through dramatically different landscape to the Blue City. Jodhpur is blue, the way the Blue Mountains are, more so from a distance. We drive through desert country—long, wide expanses of sand, with mountains in the distance—into the middle of town. We follow trucks with brightly colored murals painted on their back panels.

Mahendra explains things we are longing to understand; and we try to catch all we can from his broken English. We pass camels in the street, elephants, pigs and piglets, women in bold colored saris, palm trees and cactus-like plants. Jodhpur is more than blue; it is every bit as colorful as I imagine Mexican and South American cities to be.

We pull up to a sprawling oasis that turns out to be the hotel Mahendra has chosen for us. A man helps with our bag and we follow. Mahendra calls to us that he will be back soon. What a difference it makes learning to trust people completely. We arrive in the middle of a desert without buying plane tickets ourselves, without knowing if we will stay with Mahendra or somewhere else, without return tickets to leave here, with no idea of the name of Mahendra's factory, where he lives, or when he'll be back. We simply follow the man who carries our bag and the key to our room.

We turn on the overhead fan; the combination of the fan's clicking and the heat reminds me of the old farmhouse in the Florida swamp in the movie *Cross Creek*, about the writer Marjorie Rawlings. The furniture is rattan; the shower is tile and without a curtain. There is a water-holding tank that I wonder if we will be able to figure out how to heat. I pick up an extra roll of toilet paper, but need my glasses to read the print on it.

"We don't know how long we have before he returns," I say coming out of the bathroom, "so why...." Howard is already lying down on the bed, his mouth open slightly, whispering sleep straight up into the air like tiny bubbles.

The toilet paper is wrapped in an orange label that says MAPLE™ Toilet Tissues, made from Imported PULP—the "pulp" part in all caps. Over a white maple leaf that I can associate only with Canada is the slogan "Relation of Love, Care & Hygiene." On the back side of the wrapping, I read that it is manufactured by Purple Paper Products in India, and claims to be "mellow to skin, super absorbent and Eco friendly" among many other admirable qualities.

I think of all the places I have traveled, and consider the possibility of starting a toilet tissue study. When I was in London I remember having to pay the water-closet attendant ten pence to buy a square of toilet paper that felt like onionskin stationery. In my study, I will compare not only the texture and durability of the tissue itself, but also brand names and slogans. I remove the wrapper, fold it, and stuff it inside the zipper pocket of my pack. It takes only two to start a collection. I will be on the lookout for more.

Mahendra calls from the lobby, the lobby we haven't seen yet. We assume he has come to take us with him, so we get ready and step outside. He is waiting by his car right where we pulled in. The other man is no longer with him. Mahendra drives us through Jodhpur again. When we pull up alongside a camel at a red light, I am giddy.

We drive out into the desert again to Lakeview, a lovely resort on a reservoir. We park and walk across a long bridge over a tip of the lake and sandy rocks to the restaurant that overlooks the water. We are the only people here, I assume because it is midday. Wild monkeys, the color of light caramel, with whips for tails, are the ones most excited to see us.

Inside the resort, we meet an Italian couple. Apparently, they are friends of Mahendra's, a young man and an older woman. Mahendra leads us to a side room off the main dining area with many fans whirring and a long low table between two sofas. We are to have dinner with these two Italians who are here to buy furniture from Mahendra's factory.

The Italians do not speak English, and we do not speak Italian. Mahendra speaks a tiny bit of each, so it is hard work for all of us to communicate. We manage to get the basic introduction of why each of us is here, but are glad for the food that Mahendra orders: the sizzler sampler, dal and soup and beer. It provides a welcome diversion for us all.

I can see Howard is tiring in this heat. He hasn't had a real nap yet today, and we have flown across part of India. But I'm sure he is thrilled to be somewhere besides Delhi.

After the awkward but generous meal and some difficult conversation, even the Italians are tired. Mahendra takes us to his factory, and we learn later that the Italians have gone back to their room for a nap. Mahendra explains their absence in a somewhat jumbled explanation: it sounds as though part of their buying trip involved drinking long into the night, after dinner yesterday.

When we step out of Mahendra's car, a young man and woman approach us and put leis around our necks. They are fresh and fragrant strings of orange marigolds and red roses. Queen and King for a day! The furniture factory sits behind chain-link fencing and seems to sprawl on and on, a building here, an open-to-the-sky workspace there, another warehouse over there.

We wander, looking at the furniture, most of it hefty and intricately carved like the furniture you might find at Pier 1 Imports, or Cost Plus in San Francisco. Howard is intrigued by the number of young men working on large pieces of furniture in the dirt outside. They use mostly hand tools, and they sand and chisel to make things fit.

"There are so many of them," Howard says.

"They are so young," I say. The boys seem to range in age from ten to maybe twenty. They watch us as we tour the facility with Mahendra. Everyone must think we are here as buyers, choosing furniture to order and have delivered in large cartons on ships. Neil, Howard's Swedish friend, comes here as well as to North Carolina to buy furniture for his store in Sweden. He told us he orders furniture at the furniture shows, then waits many months to receive the shipment. Neil also described how quickly they can sell the large cartons full of sofas, tables, chairs back in Sweden.

The workers are every bit as fascinating to me as the furniture, especially since we aren't here to buy any furniture. One boy turns on a shower on the side of the first building and rinses himself off. Rats scurry across the back fence. Under one shelter, several boys sit in the dirt around a fire they have built. They are patting dough into flat circles. They must be making roti, the bread I ate with each meal in the hospital. No one actually explains this to us, but it is obvious that these boys live here.

They cook, shower, and work, probably around the clock, behind a locked fence, safe from whatever other boys their age in town might be vulnerable to. They must not get paid much, but they have a life that includes work and food and shelter. I think of the Light Child from the park. I doubt he has this much. He has become a part of me. I see him everywhere.

We sit with Mahendra in another office, and a woman brings us sweets and bottled water. He shows us three-ring binders filled with furniture photos. I feel as though we've misled someone—at the least the woman who serves us, possibly Mahendra too. We don't know what Neil has told him about us. But we are in no position to buy even a small table, let alone cartons of furniture to ship home. We ask him about the workers as we flip through the pages of photographs.

Mahendra tells us that he has more than one hundred employees now. The sky darkens and the boys still work.

Another one showers. More gather around the fire. Several groups of workers are still planing the ends of tables, and sanding chair legs. Mahendra finally asks if we are ready to go back to our room.

We agree. We are tired and need to rest. As he drives, he asks if we would like for him to come back and pick us up for dinner later, to party with his Italian friends. I'm delighted when Howard says, "I think I am ready for bed."

Mahendra is noticeably surprised, maybe even disappointed. My guess is that he feels obligated to show us a good time, not that we are truly fun people to hang out with. This communication thing is strenuous work, and it is really up to him with everyone who visits his factory.

I use the universal folded-hands-against-cheek gesture to explain to Mahendra that it has been a long day, and we are tired. I say, "When you come to the U.S., we will be strong and healthy, and we will party with you." I hope he understands. I hope I am not just making small talk.

Wednesday, October 20, 2004

In the morning, we shower and pack up our things and sit on the veranda of this desert plantation. I ask for coffee. A man in a turban brings it, then asks if I will take his picture. Of course, all of this is communicated with hand signals and smiles. Being in India gives the phrase "body language" new significance. Mahendra pulls up in his SUV and joins us on the patio.

He has sacks of gifts for us: several boxes of Jodhpur sweets for us to take back to the U.S. for our party, bags of snack mix. Then he presents me with a tiny box. I open it to find a beautiful ring with an elliptical setting of stones that at least look like diamonds and amethysts. Inscribed in the band it says 23K. I try it on and it fits! Is this man not only kind and generous beyond belief, but also a sage?

"How did you know my size?"

"I know," he says, trying not to smile.

"It is beautiful, Mahendra." And I get up to hug him. "Thank you so much."

"You must not thank me," he says again. "You are my guest. This is my country." He says this with such earnestness, it sounds more like personal doctrine than spontaneous affection.

"So when you visit me, I must buy you a ring?" I ask.

He finally smiles. Understanding joking is one of the true signs of successful communicating, someone once told me.

Mahendra picks up our bag and we load ourselves back into the car. We drive without much conversation through this festive town of bright colors. Storefronts are painted with murals, women wear saris of every imaginable color. Trucks are painted with slogans and pictures. I take snapshots of camels and elephants stopped in traffic before we head out into the desert again.

We pass an enormous estate, an elaborate building. "This is the Palace," Mahendra says. "Do you want to go inside?"

"No, this is good," Howard says. Mahendra explains that this palace was built during a famine in order to provide employment for the workers. We keep driving, heading toward a hillside on the horizon. As we approach, we can see an old terraced castle perched way up on a high hill. "This is Mehrangarh Fort," Mahendra says.

"Is it named after you?" I ask. No response.

He drives up the steep road, past women in colorful costumes. All the color against the drab sand and rock makes me smile.

"Is this a holiday?" I ask. "Everyone is so dressed up."

"This is normal dress for Jodhpur," Mahendra replies. He parks the car and says, "I wait here."

"No, please come with us," I say. I want him to be our friend, not our tour guide.

He shakes his head, "Thieves steal bags in cars. I wait for you."

So Howard and I climb the steep hill to the entrance. It is a workout for anyone in this heat, let alone someone with a brand-new heart valve. The fortress is a stunning example of ancient architecture, with exquisitely carved panels, lattice windows, and narrow passageways, yet the people here are citizens of the twenty-first century. We pass a platform where a woman and a man sell water in old clay urns. They are filled from an underground spring.

Shrines have been carved into the walls of this fortress; dozens of tiny rooms nested among the rocks. I have no way to judge if they are personal memorials or communal altars decorated by anyone. Candles are lit. Incense is burning. I drop coins onto one altar, my lei onto another and each time, say a silent prayer for Howard's heart.

I am grateful for the opportunity to see as a tourist sees, and to ask for healing in this ancient, holy place. Out of our sight, someone is singing, not with words but a beautiful high-pitched chant. The song of angels. We follow the music until we see two young boys in bright orange and red garments, sitting on the ground singing; they're playing instruments we will never be able to name. Their song is one of the most exhilarating and, at the same time, soothing blends of voices and strings I've ever heard. We stop to listen. Howard closes his eyes. I toss coins into the basket beside them.

I don't want to leave, but it is hot, we are thirsty, and Howard hasn't eaten yet. "Ready?" I ask. He nods.

Slowly, we make our way down the hill to where Mahendra is parked. He is standing outside the car in this intense sun, the same way Rajul, our driver at the hotel, waits for us while we shop or eat. "I tell the truth," he says.

"What?" I ask.

He explains that a man tried to break into the back of his car to steal our bags. "He does not see me in the front seat." Mahendra laughs. I cringe—a seat away from a burglary.

"Thank you for saving us, again," I say.

"Now we must go," he says, looking at his cell phone for the time.

Mahendra drives toward the airport, but decides we have time to stop to eat.

He picks a restaurant where we can get *dosas*, the thin crepes or pancakes only one Indian restaurant at home serves. We have wanted to try them here in India. Inside, the lights are off. The high-backed booths are made of dark wood. Ceiling fans click in their lazy spinning, but don't offer much relief from the heat. We slip into a booth, Howard and me on one side, Mahendra facing us. He orders for us again, which speeds up the process tenfold.

Howard is quiet, listless, and when he reaches for my hand under the table his is clammy. I count this as fatigue, overheating, and lack of food. He will bounce back as soon as we drink some water and eat this dosa. As it turns out, Mahendra orders three dosas; each one completely covers a dinner plate. The food is wonderful, but quite spicy. Good for me; a challenge for Howard just now, I am sure. As we eat, I try to make simple conversation, which I presume is as tiring for Mahendra as it is for us.

No one wants just to sit and look at people they're supposed to like, but cannot talk to. I realize I've no idea whether he is married, has children, what he loves besides his successful furniture factory. I don't even know if he is in his thirties, forties, or fifties. He checks the time on his cell phone and says, "We must go to airport."

Howard starts to scoot out of the booth first, but stumbles. Mahendra grabs his arm. I slide out and grab his other arm. Howard is melting. His face is pouring sweat and he is the color of white ash. We get him into the car. He slumps deeply into the seat. Something is wrong—terribly wrong.

At the airport, I tell Mahendra we need a wheelchair. He tells an attendant, we load up our bags, and say goodbye to our new friend. I push Howard into the terminal, his head hanging down to one side. I am on my own again, with a collapsed Howard. Only this time, we are boarding an airplane.

In the terminal, we wait. We wait some more. I have to make several trips to the bathroom, and Howard is slumped over, asleep in the wheelchair. The plane is not here, we are not allowed to move into the gate area. No one tells us why our flight is late. It is hot, even with fans blowing. It is the kind of heat that makes me want to just close my eyes and fall into a deep, drugged sleep. The kind of sleep where I will dream about water, maybe a waterfall, or crashing waves.

Somehow, in the long, slow blur of this afternoon, I finally jockey Howard in his wheelchair through Security. The guards insist that I open the Jodhpur sweets and reveal the entire contents of our bag. The small plane has finally arrived, and we board.

In Delhi, we exit and find another wheelchair. A man holds a sign with Howard's name printed on it. Déjà vu. The man is Raj's driver. Apparently, Mahendra has called ahead to Raj and asked him to send someone to pick us up. I am beyond grateful. What would I do? In silence, he loads us into his car and drives us back to the Centrum Hotel. He refuses our money. Raj must pay him a regular wage for his services, no matter what he asks him to do.

When the desk clerks at the Centrum see us pull up, I watch their welcoming smiles turn to alarm when they see Howard get out of the car. They rush out to help me get him inside and up to our room. I turn on the air-conditioning as soon as Howard is flat on the bed. I don't understand.

I long to be able to name these events he experiences. I never know what to expect. I am told not to worry. I am told his recovery is proceeding normally. I keep wondering whether we will be told the same thing at home ... if we make it back. One thing I am sure of: Howard will not be seeing the Taj Mahal, unless of course, he can get his crew to move it to the park just down the street.

Later that evening, Howard has rested and revived a bit and we discuss Agra. He agrees that the trip by car is more than he wants to try, "no matter how much gold the guy used to build the Taj." We look at the picture of the Taj Mahal in the travel book, and Howard isn't sure he would even be able to walk up the steps to see it once we got there.

We opt to stay in Delhi, maybe see the Lotus Temple together, take it easy. I call Naruna and tell him we won't be making the trip to Agra. I can't tell if he is upset or not, but again, I am clear on where my loyalty lies.

Thursday, October 21, 2004

After a good breakfast and a nap, Howard is back to his recovering self—tired, but ready to venture outside. We get a rickshaw to Escorts to deliver the last of the photos I had copied of Dr. Echo and some of the sisters. As we get back into the elevator to leave the fourth floor, Sumitra is going home.

"Do you have time to eat lunch with us?" I ask. She nods and leads us to the hospital cafeteria I knew must be here somewhere. It's where I intended to bring Howard after the Lodi Gardens fiasco. We've never eaten here. She helps us order and we sit with her looking out a window at the Lotus Temple.

"We go there today," I say.

She turns around to get a better view of the Temple, then says, "I go too."

Sumitra takes charge. She leads us out into the street, calls a rickshaw, negotiates the price to take us to the Lotus Temple, and climbs in with us. I don't understand much except that she gives us her entire afternoon. She helps us understand the procedures at the Temple: navigates the long lines, tells the guard Howard is a patient, shows us where to remove our shoes, and finds a seat for us inside the Temple.

The building is gorgeous with reflecting pools flanking the huge cantilevered petals that form this spectacular lotus blossom. Entering the building feels like crawling inside a Georgia O'Keeffe flower. We are finally acting like tourists seeing a Delhi attraction, and the crowds seem quite aware of that. The line is single file and slow.

I pray I won't need a bathroom. I pray Howard doesn't collapse. We make it through the entire Temple and back, and put on our shoes. We follow Sumitra out to the street and she flags down another rickshaw. She rides all the way with us back to our hotel, and then catches her bus home from there. What a gift she is. I don't know if I could have managed it all myself.

"Dhanyawaad, dhanyawaad," I call after her. "Kal malenge, dear friend."

She turns around. "Kal malenge? Yes?" She looks so happy at the idea of seeing us again tomorrow. I run over to her.

"I hope so," I say. I hug her to me. "Namaste."

I wish I knew more Hindi to tell her how much she means to me. But I can only watch her run across the street. She stops to wave two more times. She knows this is good-bye.

Friday, October 22, 2004

In the morning, we get a call from Abhay, the reporter from *Bloomberg Magazine*, who spoke with me at the press conference. He asks if he can come by to interview us one last time before we leave. Of course.

His photographer comes too, and takes pictures of us with our bags packed, ready to go. We spend a delightful day with Abhay; an easy, interesting off-the-record day. He is articulate and friendly; his English is fluid. We discuss the differences between Sikhs and Hindus and Muslims, which Howard and I have been trying to understand ever since we got here.

Abhay explains that the turbans are worn by Sikhs, and how his hair was once very long. He tells us about his wife and child who are out of town. He explains the evolution of Bloomberg's enterprises, and then offers to drop us off at Escorts to return Howard's heart monitor. When we stop in front of the guard entrance, he asks if he can take us to lunch when we are finished at Escorts.

He waits for us, and then he drives us to a wonderful Thai restaurant on the back side of the Community Center near our hotel. He helps us order. It is one of the most delicious meals we've had in India, and it's truly relaxing to be in his company.

I wouldn't mind spending the evening with him, too, but Howard needs a nap after lunch. It's difficult asking people to wait while Howard naps, but if I did ask Abhay, I think he might even do it, and graciously at that. We say good-bye to this warm man who feels almost as close a friend as Dr. Srivastava is.

The front page of today's morning newspaper has a big picture from last year's annual *Dussehra* festival. Our servers in the breakfast room point to the photo, and then to somewhere outside, away from the hotel. All I understand for sure is that the festival is today at six o'clock. The caption in the paper includes the word "Hindu," so I assume the sisters who are Christians will not be there.

I find out from the desk clerk in the hotel lobby that the festival will take place tonight at the park down the street. Howard and I agree that attending the festival will be an excellent way to spend our last evening before we head to the airport to catch our midnight flight.

We watch. We don't understand the festival or anything the speakers say, but it is thrilling to stand in this park among thousands of Indians who cheer and sing songs together. In the center of the park, three giant wood statues tower high above the crowd, propped up with wires and boards, bales of hay piled beneath them.

The best story I can come up with is that these statues are three renditions of a devil figure. The leaders with microphones call out, and the audience answers—call-and-response like in a Baptist church service. One at a time, each statue is set on fire with flames shot from a distance. One at a time, each pops and explodes and then burns like a witch at the stake. Children straddling their parents' shoulders cheer with the loss of each limb; even louder when the head topples. A good versus evil story, on a grand scale.

Finally, a huge display of fireworks lights up the sky, and Howard and I make a run for the fence. We spill out into the flood of traffic going back to our hotel, and even get lucky finding an empty rickshaw. Fireworks seem an appropriate finale.

Back in our room, we prepare envelopes of cash to leave as gifts for all the staff at the Centrum, including Rajul, the driver. We leave extra clothes and gifts of food for them to share. We arrange a cab to the airport, give hugs all around, and roll our bags across the lobby. We have been gone one month, and leaving Delhi, as with most everything these days, is bittersweet.

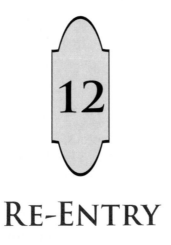

12

RE-ENTRY

Sunday, October 24, 2004

Our plane lands over a thick blanket of green treetops and the winding ropes of interstates and roads we recognize. Howard and I sit forward in our seats; I can sense we are both trying to squelch our excitement. I wonder if Howard can hear his heartbeat from right there in his seat.

The flight attendant leans down over Howard. "If you will stay seated and allow the other passengers to deplane, we will have your wheelchair for you in a minute."

"Thank you," I say.

When the attendant turns around, Howard looks at me. "I'm walking."

And so he does. Off the plane, past the attendant who thinks he needs a wheelchair, from the gate all the way out to where my parents are waiting for us, just beyond the security checkpoint.

We are home.

We must wait for baggage, but we do not wait alone or silently. We wait chitchatting with my mother and father. They know us, they love us. They laugh and speak English. Never have I been so comforted to see them. The most pressing decision I must make is how to keep everyone from carrying our bags. Who is less able to carry them? Howard who's just had heart surgery, my father who has severe back problems, or my eighty-year-old mother who is facing knee (maybe both knees), and possibly hip, replacements in the coming year?

I insist on a luggage cart to avoid the discussion. Once we are loaded in the car, my father drives their smooth silver Honda out the airport exit onto I-40. There are thick stands of pine trees and grassy medians planted with flowers along most of the highway. When we exit, there are streetlights, bushes, trees turning amber and red, sidewalks, porch lights, mailboxes, and driveways on the sides of the road. There are edges here! Everything is wide enough to have borders.

In Delhi, the people and animals and campfires and store-fronts and vendors' carts and food and clothes-for-sale and butchers' blocks and cages of chickens and garbage and water running down the street are all woven together. Howard could never estimate the width of a Delhi street, because it is impossible to tell where one starts and stops. There are no curbs; there are no edges. In fact, outside of Escorts Heart Institute, there are few boundaries of any kind. "Organized chaos," I think Bryan called it.

Dad coasts down the gentle hill that leads to Howard's house. I hope Howard's body is relaxing the way mine is. No need to be on guard. We are safe. We are home. Howard is alive. I hope he is paying attention. But he is making jokes with my father, promising my mother a game of Scrabble as soon as we get a good night's sleep.

We pull into Howard's driveway, past his mailbox with the flying hammer logo on it. Even the sound of the gravel crunching under my father's tires is soothing. Howard's house, newly painted Outgoing Orange and Mediterranean Blue, clearly match his new outfit from Fab India. Even on this clear autumn evening, I can imagine the sound of rain on his new tin roof. I repeat the words the sister taught me to say for "it is raining"—"barish ho rahi hai." I hope I can remember it by the time it rains again here.

Over the next several days, Howard and I try to reconnect to this uncluttered life we almost managed to forget. We visit with a few friends who stop by, call others on the phone, e-mail even more. We open cards from people who found out about Howard after we were gone. I try to organize our photos so we can show people our story instead of trying to tell it over and over.

We feel the weight of our journey, the sheer magnitude of all we do not yet realize we have learned. India has moved in and taken over my consciousness. I wear a bindhi every day. Howard and I rest a lot in between routine chores of resuming housekeeping—laundry, tending the garden, feeding his cats—and of retelling our story to anyone who asks. Howard's crew works in his shop. I can see Howard's longing to join them. But he is operating at slow speed.

Possibly because we are both so relieved to have something to focus on other than Howard's heart, neither of us mentions seeing Dr. Engel. One evening while I'm putting away the medical files we've brought home, I say, "I guess we should go see Dr. Engel sometime."

Howard looks up. "Yeah, weren't we supposed to contact her as soon as we got home?"

"I don't remember that. But I'll call the office and leave a message telling her we are back."

The next day, Dr. Engel's nurse returns my call. She schedules an appointment for Howard to see Dr. Engel in a few days. Meanwhile, the reporters who interviewed us before we left for India call asking to do follow-up interviews. At the suggestion of the reporter from the *Raleigh News and Observer*, Vicki, we agree to let her accompany us to Howard's appointment with Dr. Engel on Tuesday. She will get the appropriate permission. We will meet her there.

Vicki brings a photographer with her on Tuesday. All four of us are in the room when Dr. Engel comes in. We give her a box of sweets from Jodhpur and the best souvenir of all—a smiling Howard.

Dr. Engel admires Howard's color and overall physical condition. She asks him to remove his shirt and admires his bright pink scars. She asks a lot of questions, and seems a bit surprised about his choice of the natural pig valve over the St. Jude, the mechanical valve. But she is happy about how well his wounds are healing and how strong his heart sounds.

We explain about the TIA when Howard lost his vision. She asks me if it was the only episode he had. I honestly answer that I'm not sure. I tell her about the times Howard stumbled, and about his occasional loss of right-side motor function, and speech. I tell her about him collapsing at lunch in Jodhpur. I tell her I feared the worst, but people kept telling me not to worry.

I lost confidence in my ability to discern a normal recovery course of good-days/bad-days from dangerous relapses. She looks over the thick stack of reports we've brought with us and takes a blood sample. Vicki, the photographer, and Howard and I are joking around when Dr. Engel returns.

"Your PT is way too low," Dr. Engel says. "Too low" tells me that according to the neurologist at Escorts, Howard's blood is not thin enough to prevent a stroke. "Dangerously low." She explains that given my description of Howard's episodes, she can only assume he had more clots, more ministrokes. "We have to get your blood to between a 2 and 3, or we stand a chance of you throwing a clot that will lodge somewhere and cause permanent damage. That is not a risk worth taking."

"Why is it too low?" I ask. "Is it the warf we got in India?" I think of the fake seal on the bottle of water, and then how the chemist showed me the seal and date on the foil pack of Howard's warfarin.

"When is the last time your blood was checked over there?" Dr. Engel asks.

Howard and I look at each other. I can't remember, and neither of us can come up with an exact date.

"They seemed to stick him every time we went to Escorts," I say. But we hadn't been back since at least two weeks ago by now, except the time we went to return Howard's heart monitor. I doubt they checked it then.

"People who begin on Coumadin or its generic, warfarin, must be continually checked to keep the levels in check. Everything you eat and drink affects it. And you haven't been seen by any doctor in over two weeks. Anything could be making it low right now. We just need to get it back on track."

"So should he take two warfarins?" I ask. I remember how scared I was when I gave him a whole tablet instead of a half.

Dr. Engel shakes her head. I can tell our celebration is over.

"Oral blood thinners like Coumadin won't work fast enough," she explains. "Howard needs heparin. Intravenously. And the only way to get it is in the hospital."

I feel myself putting on the armor of stoicism again, leg by leg, arm by arm, and then, when my eyes feel so hot they might ignite, I pull down my face mask. I will not cry.

"How long?" Howard asks.

"Two days." Dr. Engel promises to try everything she can do to admit him just for the heparin, without any other tests or services. "I'm sorry," she says. "I wish there was a way to administer it at home." She looks down at Howard's chart. She knows what this means to us.

"Two days will cost us what the entire month cost in India," Howard says.

"I'll do everything I can," she says. "There's no alternative that is worth the risk of a clot."

Howard will not look at me. I reach out to touch his shoulder. "We just do it," I say. "We just do it." He pulls away and puts on his shirt.

The photographer has already excused himself, and I'm sure Vicki wishes she left with him. This is not the party we thought it would be. Howard and I go directly to Durham Regional Hospital for two days of heparin drip to prevent any trouble with clots. It feels like complete sacrilege to park in the same parking lot we parked in to visit the CFO two months ago now, begging to be allowed to pay what insurance companies pay. Once assigned a hospital room, I settle myself in the chair beside Howard. If I learned anything in

India, it is that we can do this. I pick up the phone and begin to call all the people who need to know we won't be coming back home.

A nurse comes in to start the IV drip. I don't even want to look at Howard's face. I'm afraid we will both start crying, and I can't predict who will be first.

Howard is irritable with me. He tells me to go home. Hot off the plane, I am supposed to go home and leave him here, in this hospital, now that I'm off duty? Now that my services are no longer needed? We sit in silence. He turns on the TV. A meal tray comes and once he sees it, he covers it back up.

"I can go get us pizza," I say. "You're allowed to eat anything while you're on blood thinners except tomatoes and spinach and stuff high in Vitamin K. Remember what they—"

"I'm not sick," he shouts. "You don't need to sleep in that chair. Go home. I can do this myself."

"I haven't even been to my own home," I say. "My cats aren't even there yet." We argue. Then we opt for a painful silence. I should leave. But I don't dare. A nurse brings in a toothbrush.

"How much extra does that cost?" I ask.

"Oh, nothing. It's all included." "Included" is the operative word. She has no idea.

The nurse goes to the mirror over Howard's sink and puts on mascara and eye liner. I try to imagine one of the sisters doing that at Escorts. I walk down to the nurses' station and ask about ice and water. A nurse points to the ice room down the hall. I fill a pitcher, get cups, and grab a pillow from an unoccupied room for myself. Somehow we manage to sleep until Dr. Engel comes by in the morning.

"You are not sick," she says, then turns to me. "Don't act like he's sick. He can walk around. He doesn't have to stay in bed. He can eat anything he wants to eat; we just have to get this heparin in him." I don't argue with her. I don't tell her I was the one who suggested pizza last night.

Vicki, the only reporter who knows we are here, calls to ask if it is a good day to come for a visit. She wants to ask about the difference in care between Escorts and Durham Regional Hospital. When she arrives, she finds us down the hall in the waiting room visiting with my parents, playing a game of Scrabble.

Vicki asks us if we know what this will cost. Of course, that will make the best lead for a follow-up story, and of course, it will be weeks before we know.

Later that evening, no one comes to clean the room, and the blood from the first heparin stick still stains Howard's sheets. No one has mentioned bathing. I walk down to the nurses' station and ask if I can get sheets out of the linen closet to change Howard's bed. The nurse sitting at the station reading a book looks up and says, "Sure, go ahead," then realizes she must open the door with a combination code.

She gets up, hands me the sheets, and goes back to her book. I change Howard's bed while he is visiting with his friend Will. I get more ice in the pitcher. I do a cross-word puzzle that my parents brought for me yesterday. The silence is excruciating. These two days are longer than any at Escorts, even the last two days when he was receiving the heparin drip there.

The following morning, Dr. Engel's assistant comes to discharge Howard. His blood work shows he is up to 2.3, and he can go home. But they are changing his prescription from warfarin to Coumadin, and Howard is instructed to return to get his blood checked in two days. I deliver him back to his house, pick up my cats from Susan's house, and begin my own re-entry into my home only a few miles away.

My parents checked on my house once a week while we were gone. When my father smelled how musty it was becoming in my basement studio, he plugged in the old dehumidifier I took home from their moving sale in September. But my house has been shut up, without air-conditioning, for the entire month of October. I open the screen door, open the windows, but I begin to sneeze and cough almost immediately.

I discover that while I was gone, blue mold moved in. I clean furniture and clothes and linens, wipe down counters and walls and floors. I open closets and start a sneezing fit that burns through my eyes until they are tiny red slits. Finally, I realize everything I own is moldy. I remove coats and wash dozens of loads of clothes and hang them on the line. One day I pick a shoe box for a pair of closed shoes instead of the sandals I've worn since June. The shoes are covered in blue mold.

I haul outside every pair of shoes, every belt and purse, and stack them on my porch. Since I worked in a shoe store when I was sixteen, I've always loved shoes. At any given point in my life, I've owned more shoes than dishes. I face a monumental task of cleaning my belongings. I take carloads to the thrift shop, garbage sacks to the dump, sneezing the entire way, with tears and itchy eyes. This is not how I planned to resume my life. I am just plain sick, and Howard is sick of me.

One afternoon I hear what at first I think are cicadas or a band of crickets in the trees. Then the tap-tap-clicking speeds up, as if someone is cranking up an old gramophone to recognize the song. It is the neighbor boy who learned to ride a bike last spring, speeding past my house. As he nears my yard, the sound becomes louder and faster. He has playing cards fastened to his spokes with clothespins.

My first thought is of how my brothers and sisters and I also used cards to make our bikes look cool. My second thought is of the children in Delhi. They would never think of this way to spruce up their bikes, even if they had the cards. They would never be able to hear the sound over the constant honking and clattering in the streets. Besides, where would they ride without edges to their streets?

Howard meets with a few clients who had agreed to wait for his return, and soon he is back on the job site, ordering supplies and designing cabinets for his crew. Reporters e-mail and call. Howard wants nothing to do with any of it. He wants to put India, and apparently his heart too, behind him. I, however, feel an urgent need to respond to the public's interest in Howard's story, hoping it might help other people to learn there are alternatives to our own broken health care system. I take on the task, instead of letting it drop. Tim Nelson, from Channel 11 news, interviews us again.

Everywhere we go, people stare. At first, we think it is just coincidence. Then, enough people stop to speak to us, to tell us they saw us on the news, that we finally realize Howard's face is now a public one. We seem to be drawn to grocery store checkout lines with Indian cashiers. We ask where they are from. Mumbai, Goa, Chennai, many of the cities we thought we would visit. Every Indian clerk catches my eye, as if I had never seen one before our trip. I am drawn to these people, and seeing them makes me homesick for the fourth floor. It is ridiculous, and I know it. I try to re-create their accents so I can hear the sisters' voices, Dr. Trehan's, Naruna's and Sanjiv's. All I see are their smiling, generous faces. I hope I never forget.

We hear from people all over the States with mitral valve problems, wanting to know what to do. We are bombarded with reporters who want to do follow-up stories that include other Americans who are on their way to Escorts. We were the first. I know of no one else who is going—yet. After at least a dozen people ask us to send them the names and phone numbers of some other Americans who have decided on India, I scream at my computer screen. "Do your own homework!" (As if I would forward a list of people with heart disease who are sick enough and desperate enough to contact me, a perfect stranger, for advice.)

One evening while we are walking in Duke Forest I ask Howard, "Have you heard from your sister?" The forest is one of our favorite places to catch up on each other's day.

"Not since before India," Howard says.

I can tell this is not the first time he has realized the lack of a response from his only remaining family.

"She hasn't called or e-mailed," he says. "Nothing."

"Do you feel like calling her?" I ask, kicking up some leaves, hoping to keep this light.

"Yes and no. Remember when I called her to tell her about my diagnosis?"

Of course I remember. Isn't it just like a sibling you hoped would be supportive to ridicule your decision? And she did. "Wasn't it an I-told-you-so speech about your not having health insurance?" I ask, as if I could forget that blow to Howard.

"Yep." Howard doesn't look at me. "She's either pissed off or out of the country."

"So why not call her? Maybe she's waiting for you to call."

Howard calls her later in the week. When he finally tells me about their conversation, I can hardly believe it.

"She told me how wrong it was for me to take other people's money when it was my decision not to have insurance," he says. "She says she is embarrassed and angry. One more time, she thinks I am a bad person."

"Because of Howard's Heart Fund?" I ask.

Howard nods.

"We didn't coerce anyone to donate money." I can't believe that after fighting for Howard's life, we are expected to apologize for offering tangible answers to the question "How can I help?"

"Does she know we started that back when we thought you were going to have to come up with $200,000? Does she know it still cost lots of money for both of us to be off work for close to three months, and to live in India for a month?" I feel the heat rising in my cheeks. "Did you tell her you gave a child the gift of heart surgery?" I haven't lost it for some time, maybe since the rickshaw driver took us so far out of our way. But I feel out of control. I know the correct answer is to ignore Howard's sister. But there's something about family crises that still reaches a raw spot. I know from my own personal crisis over a decade ago that the disapproval of a sibling is a thousand times more hurtful than that of a stranger.

We continue to hear from people who have no insurance, who have heart disease, who need dental work, who are dying and want to go to India. Students call for information for their dissertations on health care. A friend calls to tell us that he had to be admitted to the same hospital in Durham for IV antibiotics when his tooth abscessed. He just received his bill for $7,500 for one night's hospital stay; more than Howard's entire Escorts' bill. Entrepreneurs, eager to capitalize on this new way of outsourcing medical care, call and write to us. I ignore most of them. Then a former hospital

CEO and his Indian friend contact us. They are hoping to form a partnership with Escorts to help people from the U.S. get to India for surgery. They invite us to dinner to pick our brains. We dine and let them pick away.

It is invigorating to retell the story of the expertise and generosity of all the people involved with Howard's care. And now, with a real sense of the sheer number of people interested in obtaining medical care in India who don't know where to begin, we recognize the need for someone to serve as liaison. However, we are cautious in our enthusiasm. "We only want to make sure your middleman role doesn't make it unaffordable for those who really need to go," I say to the CEO and his Indian friend before we say good night. One day, I get an e-mail from a reporter from *The NewsHour with Jim Lehrer* on PBS. I'd done a telephone interview with her before we left, when Howard didn't have the strength to talk to her.

"I wrote a piece on covering the uninsured that mentioned the *Washington Post's* story on Howard's surgery," she writes. "I'm following up now because I've received a letter from a doctor in Massachusetts who is asserting some things about the alleged inferior quality of care Howard received in India. I don't know what to make of these allegations but I wanted to talk things over with you and Howard to see if we can shed light on why this doctor feels this way."

Inferior quality of care? I am stunned. What possible basis would a doctor in Massachusetts have to say this? If he had been there, he certainly failed to introduce himself to us. I ask the reporter for a copy of the letter. This U.S. doctor has made a public claim to Howard's inferior care and to his poor prognosis because he didn't have his valve repaired by the expert at Duke University. I have no idea why anyone, especially this doctor, would find some benefit in suggesting this after the fact.

Moreover, the care was comprehensive, immediate, and delivered with compassion and genuine kindness. Howard had absolutely no pain from the surgery throughout the entire ordeal, except for the 1 A.M. gastritis episode, and of course, when he tried to climb on top of me in my bed and fell on the floor. I am speechless—almost speechless. I try my best to respond with accurate medical information that I learned from Dr. Trehan and Dr. Echo. I ask the reporter to get in touch with Dr. Engel to make sure I have it right.

A woman from CNN in New York calls—they are doing a story in conjunction with an upcoming trip to visit several private hospitals in India. I urge her to be patient in India; people are generous but things take place on a different timetable. I suggest she might want to get in touch with Suhasini from CNN in Delhi since her multiple interviews with us have not yet turned into a story. CNN from DC airs a brief piece on the Howard's Heart Web site, which is picked up and aired on local news channels.

I finally hear from Suhasini that her story has been cut, due to other more pressing issues, including our presidential elections, and then the tsunami that struck southern India. I get a taste of the work reporters put into a story that may never even see the cutting room door, let alone the floor.

The television show 60 Minutes calls. Howard talks with the reporter, and then I talk with him for quite a while, too. They too are traveling to India to cover this hot topic: the outsourcing of medical care from the U.S. As usual, the reporter wants to know the names of other patients going to India. I explain that they will have to find them. I do give him names of people to talk to at Escorts who speak very fluent

English. The reporter promises to fly us to New York City for a personal interview when he returns from Delhi.

Many weeks later, Howard gets an e-mail from the same reporter telling us the story will air Sunday night. Not only is Howard's story not included, but the 60 *Minutes* piece is watered down to reflect nothing of the fortitude it takes to get there, and talks more about cosmetic surgery and hip replacement than life-threatening situations. We are disappointed that the reporters keep missing the point. Why did we choose to go to India? Not to sit on the beach at Goa after a tummy tuck.

What is wrong with our health care system that makes no provision for people without insurance? What is wrong with our health insurance system that prevents insurance companies from paying for the immunizations and inoculations I needed for safe travel to India? What about the prevention of malaria, typhoid, polio, and hepatitis? I still don't understand why Blue Cross Blue Shield would rather pay for my health care if I had contracted one of these diseases in India than to pay for the medicine that would prevent me from becoming ill in the first place.

We contact Michael Moore, whose new documentary, we hear, is on health care and the health insurance industry. Interest concerning this issue remains high. Responding to everyone is a full-time job.

It is November and I push Howard to schedule our Dhanyawaad Party for all those who kept our children and pets, looked after our houses, mowed Howard's lawn, supervised Howard's construction jobs, brought food, and sent donations to Howard's Heart Fund. We set the date, December 6.

Tandoor Restaurant brings Indian hors d'oeuvres. Howard's friend, Jim, at J&J's Deli creates enormous submarine sandwiches, delivers them on Sunday afternoon, and then refuses to accept payment. Howard and I dress in our kurtas and pajamas and I wear my dupatta from Fab India. Even though they still carry a strong odor, I wear the red shoes the man at Central Market dunked into a bucket of dye.

We serve the Jodhpur sweets and snacks Mahendra gave us. We buy cases of mango juice and Kingfisher beer. I hire a band, but they do not show up. So Howard and I dance anyway to a CD, the way we imagined we would for the Hoe-Down fund-raiser, the way we hoped we would when we first talked about this thank-you party in Howard's hospital room in Delhi.

We set out the photo albums and notebooks filled with articles about Howard that I've gathered and assembled. We put heart stickers on each of the guests, and I offer bindhis to all the women. Some friends bring soup and cookies, and some bring additional contributions to Howard's Heart Fund which has already helped so much with the ongoing medical expenses since Howard has been away from work.

The holidays approach and my family members agree to give money to families in need this year, instead of buying senseless gifts for each other. We have so much to be thankful for, with Howard's complete recovery, and no one has to walk the streets of Delhi to realize we have all we really need. Each of my siblings chooses a different charity to give to, or picks specific needy children from Family Services or the Salvation Army.

My parents choose a Hispanic family with two very small children; their father was killed in a car accident just one month ago. I help them shop, and with an interpreter, we deliver the clothes and toys to the mother and children who speak only Spanish. My mother holds the little one in diapers on her lap and reads a book aloud. My father shows the older one how a rubber alphabet puzzle works. Later, my parents send an additional check for groceries.

Howard and Susan and I choose a family to sponsor together. We buy clothes and food and a television set. Their joy is so contagious; we choose another family and do more shopping. It is a Christmas that feels most like the way I've always wanted Christmas to feel. But when I am shopping, I cannot help wondering what size shoes the Light Child would wear.

One night at dinner, I sit with my parents and Howard and ask them what they think of the nagging voice inside me that keeps telling me to write this story.

I tell my parents that I keep hearing from people who don't think they have any choices. I even heard from Don, a friend from high school, who has been diagnosed with mitral valve disease too. He explains he is living with his heart condition untreated because he can't get health insurance. He can't afford health insurance because he doesn't have a job. And he can't get a job because of his heart condition. The U.S. health care version of Catch-22!

I want people to know they have choices. I want to include all of the information that will help people make informed decisions, prepare to go, travel safely, and return home with less distress than we experienced. The more that patients know ahead of time, the less shocking the experience will be, and the faster they will heal. It is my hope that flying to India for health care will be about a person's health, with minimal anxiety over the practical negotiations of living in a third-world country.

"Imagine if it could be easy ... and even fun," I say. We all agree. I will begin writing the story in January, after the holidays.

Howard builds a cabinet for a friend for Christmas. He regains his strength and does a few push-ups and sit-ups in the morning in addition to our frequent walks. He says he feels fine—"Not a hundred percent like you, but getting there," he says. His blood is steady at the right thinness, and he will have to be on Coumadin only for a couple of more months to ensure the valve is completely "adopted" by his own body tissue. Dr. Engel wants to make sure there will be no more clots running around loose.

There really is nothing Howard is not doing except getting up on roofs or riding his bicycle. When he is no longer on Coumadin and no longer at risk for uncontrolled bleeding, he will be able to do those things again, too. His color is good and he has regained all of the weight he lost—even a bit extra for this holiday season, like most Americans.

One evening, Howard and I walk to Akai Hana Japanese Restaurant in Carrboro. We sit at the Sushi Bar so we can watch the chefs roll and pat and decorate the platters. The server brings us menus and two hotter-than-usual white cloths on a bamboo rack. I hold the washcloth up to my face and resist pulling away from the heat. My glasses steam to opaque. When I turn to Howard, I can make out that he is still holding his washcloth to his face, but I see his upper body moving up and down.

"This reminds me of the steam," he says. My glasses clear and I see the movement is Howard breathing in deeply from the cloth. His eyes are closed. Instantly I know he is referring to the white porcelain pots of steam the sisters in India brought him every few hours. They asked him to suck the hot steam through the tube to help break up the sputum in his lungs. I remember being afraid he would suck up boiling water and scald his mouth, but he explained the tube was higher than the water level. Sucking steam was the one thing the sisters asked him to do that Howard said very little about and obeyed without a fuss. I never realized how soothing it was until now.

"Thek hai," I say, toggling my head the way the sisters did.

Howard takes away the cloth and looks at me. "What did that mean? I forget."

"Thek hai," I say again. "Fine, or all good!"

January 2005

Abhay's piece in *Bloomberg Magazine* comes out. It is a slick magazine, and includes a thorough article that is about much more than Howard. It reflects our new friend's extensive research and thorough reporting.

Within three months, Howard is back at work full-time, climbing ladders, framing houses, digging footings. One clear autumn-like January morning, I pick up my parents and take folding chairs to spend the day at Howard's job site. He is building a large second-story addition over a garage in a beautiful woodsy neighborhood near his house. He's decided that it would be most efficient to cut the rafters loose from the garage and hire a crane to raise the roof while Howard's crew builds the addition.

We watch the entire process, holding our breath while the crane lifts the roof and maneuvers it between trees like it is threading a needle, and sets it in the backyard. This is like a barn raising. My father clicks dozens of pictures. The homeowner takes a video of the entire process. This would be an amazing day to remember under any circumstances. I watch Howard in his red suspenders and tool belt run around instructing his crew, race up and down ladders, laugh, and lean against a stack of 1 x 6s to eat pizza with the crane operators. His crew prepares the new subfloor and erects new walls they have already framed on the ground. They secure everything to receive the roof again.

The moment comes when the crane swings the roof back over the new second-floor addition. Dangling midair and held by thick web straps looped through the rafters at four points, the roof begins to turn. Howard jumps up. He tosses a ladder against the garage, and scrambles up. He grabs one of the straps just before the gable hits the side of the existing house. Howard gently turns the roof back into position. The crane lowers it down like a lid on a box, and the garage is transformed into brand-new living space.

"Thek hai," I call.

Howard turns to look at me. He smiles, raises his right arm. With a funny little toggle of his head, he shouts, "Thek hai!"

Afterword

As of 2006, Howard's heart is working well. In fact, some of his friends and I think it is working overtime. He and his crew are designing and building new homes; moving and renovating homes and offices; dismantling old barns to recycle the wood; buying land, historic buildings, and even lumberyards. Howard is in such demand, he must schedule new customers' projects for nine months to a year in the future. Sometimes I ask myself if Howard's unstoppable and ever-increasing workload is an indication that he never fully grasped the intimate dance with death that I witnessed.

It is common to hear of patients who have survived dramatic medical ordeals intentionally slowing down, reassessing their workload, spending more time with their families, taking more vacations, infusing their lives with more of what they truly enjoy while minimizing the hectic and frustrating aspects of their lives. Without judgment, I must assume that Howard's fast-paced work style and the accumulations of even more responsibilities and deadlines are direct sources of the pleasure in his life. Otherwise, had I not been by his side every day in India, I could only assume that Howard and I experienced the fall of 2004 in very different places.

On the first anniversary of Howard's new heart valve, he and my younger son, Thane, and I were kayaking and hiking in Cape Breton after renovating the same cabin he and I had worked on the summer of his diagnosis. It was a perfect way to celebrate.

We continue to hear from patients with life-threatening illnesses who are uninsured. Some who do have health insurance still face larger co-pays than their entire surgery would cost in India. Patients ask their questions, and then decide to stay close to home where their families and friends can be their support system. Others follow our advice to take a companion, and then journey to India. One man with Howard's exact diagnosis finally decided to take his son with him to Escorts Heart Institute. His son kept me informed during their stay at Escorts where his father received a new mitral valve and "sipped steam" brought to him by the same sisters on the fourth floor. He is back at full-time work in the States, and feeling fine. We keep in touch by e-mail, and I am delighted when he mentions his plan for a vacation.

The opportunity to respond to so many people who discover our story on the Internet, or who recognize us from the media coverage, has kept our journey at the forefront.

I provide information and encouragement to patients with other medical and dental concerns. Some I hear from again as they make their decisions, some I do not. I continue to be deeply saddened when I learn of friends who "fall between the cracks" of the health insurance system in America, as Howard did. That is, they "make too much money" to qualify for Medicaid, but the cost of private insurance is prohibitive.

Often, those with insurance have policies that do not cover the hospitalization or nursing care they need, and they cannot afford to pay the costs out-of-pocket. Some face a situation of using up all their savings, their retirement money, and leaving their spouse and families nothing when they die. We would suggest they all go to India to get the health care they need, but some are too sick to travel. And going to India is not the right choice for everyone for a variety of reasons.

Shortly after the media onslaught covering Howard's surgery, the University of North Carolina at Chapel Hill Health Care System announced that they were considering revamping their financial assistance policies, "... especially those that deal with how uninsured patients are billed for care—under mounting pressure from regulators, politicians, consumer advocates and patients" (UNC 2005; see http:// www.roperhealth.com/?p=11).

The dogged research required to get all the pieces into place to make our journey to India was daunting, I admit. Although I never once considered stopping until we had the answers we needed to make the decision and then to get on the plane, I can understand why some people could not or would not be able to stick with it. Would I do it again? In a heartbeat! Having accompanied my parents and friends to local hospitals on numerous occasions over the past year, there has never been a question whether I will stay with them or go home. I was actually surprised at my answer the last time someone asked me why I chose to spend the nights in the recliner beside their beds: "After having been to India, I might actually leave them alone there overnight. But in our hospitals, the nursing staff is so stretched, the morale often so low, I will not leave."

For me, personally, I already anticipate the decision I might make in the future, should I require nonemergency surgery. That is, even covered by Blue Cross Blue Shield of North Carolina, I would seriously consider traveling to India, to either Escorts or Apollo Hospitals, depending on the procedure I needed.

I've come to accept the fact that fully appreciating our journey to India will be a lifelong process. In these months afterward, in this time of harvest, I do not want to miss one piece of fruit that might be hiding on the vine. As promised, "... Each person on the pilgrimage must be changed in distinct ways" (Elie 2003, prologue). Certainly, Howard and I have each been changed, and clearly, in different ways. It comes down to discovering what matters, which is neither a yes or no question, nor is there a right or wrong answer.

In Sue Monk Kidd's novel, *The Secret Life of Bees*, her character, August speaks to the young girl, Lily:

> "You know, some things don't matter that much, Lily. Like the color of a house. How big is that in the overall scheme of life? But lifting a person's heart—now, *that* matters. The whole problem with people is—"
>
> "They don't know what matters and what doesn't," I said, filling in her sentence and feeling proud of myself for doing so.
>
> "I was gonna say, The problem is they *know* what matters, but they don't *choose* it. You know how hard that is, Lily? I love May, but it was still so hard to choose Caribbean Pink. The hardest thing on earth is choosing what matters" (Kidd 2002, 147)

All any of us can hope for, I expect, is to be aware of what matters to us, and then to choose it.

I continue to stay in touch with the new friends we made in India—doctors, nurses, reporters, other patients. Their compassion continues to touch me. India, the land of contradictions. Organized chaos. A third-world country with first-world state-of-the-art medical care available for a fraction of the cost of the same procedures here in the U.S. India, where the nursing care is unmatched by any I have experienced in American hospitals—where some nurses make the equivalent of $1.38 (U.S. dollars) per hour, and care for their patients as if they made thousands. India, where the generosity of the people is palpable, in the face of poverty we will never know.

In the U.S., we often wait for a tsunami or Katrina to address the deeper connections we have to the rest of humanity. In India, those connections are exposed daily. They are raw and blinding—there is no turning away. For this gift, this vision, I will forever be grateful.

Dhanyawaad.

GLOSSARY OF
MEDICAL TERMS

Cannula: A flexible tube inserted into a vessel to either drain fluid or administer a medication. Used when a patient needs frequent venous access, to avoid eventual narrowing of the vein due to scarring. Often used as a port for repeated intravenous injections.

Chordae tendonae: The small cords that connect the edges of the heart valves to the papillary muscles—Howard's "parachute strings" that snapped.

Coumadin: A brand-name anticoagulant used to prevent and treat a thrombus or embolus. Generic form of Coumadin is called Warfarin.

CT scan: Abbreviation for computed tomography. This is a radiographic technique that selects a place in the body and blurs out structures above and below that plane, leaving a clear image of the selected anatomy.

Diverticulitis: An inflammation in the intestinal tract, especially in the colon, causing pain, fever, and occasionally peritonitis.

ECG, EKG, Electrocardiogram: A simple test that produces a graphic record of the electrical activity of the heart over time which identifies cardiac irregularities such as arrhythmias, as well as heart muscle damage.

Echocardiogram ("Echo"): An ultrasound picture of the heart that measures the size of the heart and its chambers. It shows whether the heart is beating normally and whether the valves of the heart are working properly.

Heart Port technique (intercostal technique): A surgical technique to enter the thoracic cavity through the ribs instead of having to cut through the sternum.

Heparin: Intravenous blood thinner medication. A drug injected directly into a vein that thins the blood when there is danger of clotting; an anticoagulant.

Hypercontractile left ventricle function: In Howard's case, the heart had to contract (or pump) harder than normal to send blood out of the aorta to replace the blood that had leaked back out across his mitral valve.

Keloid: A red, raised formation of fibrous scar tissue caused by excessive tissue repair in response to trauma or surgical incision.

Mitral regurgitation: The abnormal leaking of blood through the mitral valve, from the left ventricle into the left atrium of the heart.

Mitral valve: The mitral valve is sometimes also called a "parachute" valve because it is attached to a supporting ring by two long cords. It lies between the left atrium and left ventricle (main pumping chamber of the heart). This valve allows blood to flow from the left atrium into the left ventricle and then prevents the back flow of blood into the left atrium during ventricular contraction.

Mitral valve prolapse (MVP), with flailing mitral valve (MV) leaflet: MVP is the most common heart problem. With this problem, the mitral valve bulges slightly back into the left atrium when it closes, allowing blood to leak backward.

The mitral valve has two cusps/leaflets (the anteromedial leaflet and the posterolateral leaflet) that guard the opening. These valve leaflets are prevented from prolapsing or bulging into the left atrium by the action of tendons attached to the posterior surface of the valve, the chordae tendonae.

Prothrombin time (PT; Pro-time): This is a test that measures the clotting time of plasma (the liquid part of the blood). The normal range is 11 to 13.5 seconds. For a person on full anticoagulant therapy, the PT should be 2 to 3 times the laboratory "control" value.

S.A.M. (Systolic Anterior Motion) of the mitral valve: The mid-septal bulge and difference in pressure that obstructs the outflow of blood from the heart. An analogy is an open door in a drafty corridor: the door starts by moving slowly and then accelerates as it presents a greater surface area to the wind and, finally, slams shut.

Sisters: The term for nurses in India. No relationship with the Catholic church.

Sternotomy: Opening the chest by cutting the sternum.

Thrombus: A blood clot that obstructs a blood vessel or a cavity of the heart. Anticoagulants are used to prevent and treat this problem.

Transesophageal echocardiogram (TEE): During the transesophageal echocardiogram test, an ultrasound transducer (which produces high-frequency sound waves) provides pictures of the heart's valves and chambers to help the physician evaluate the pumping action of the heart. The ultrasound transducer is positioned on an endoscope (a long, thin, flexible instrument about one half inch in diameter). The endoscope is placed inside the mouth and passed into the esophagus (the "food pipe" leading from the mouth into the stomach) to provide a close look at the heart's valves and chambers without interference from the ribs or lungs. TEE assesses the overall function of the heart's chambers and valves, and can identify many types of heart disease.

Transient ischemic attack (TIA): A neurological deficit, having a vascular cause that produces stroke symptoms that resolve within twenty-four hours. TIAs and strokes have similar symptoms. TIAs do not result in any residual damage.

Valvular regurgitation: A condition in which blood leaks back in the wrong direction because one or more of the heart's valves closes improperly. The nature and severity of the leakage, in turn, may keep the heart from circulating an adequate amount of blood through the defective valve. In Howard's case, the mitral valve was affected, so the diagnosis included mitral regurgitation.

Valvular stenosis: A condition in which there is a narrowing, stiffening, thickening, fusion, or blockage of one or more valves of the heart. As a result, the defective valve can interfere with the smooth passage of blood through it.

Warfarin (Wasf): An anticoagulant (blood thinner) taken orally; generic form of Coumadin used to prevent and treat a thrombus or embolus.

GLOSSARY OF
HINDI TERMS

Barish: Rain

Barish ho rahi hai: It is raining.

Bindhi or *bindi:* A small, usually red-colored decorative marking worn in the middle of the forehead by many Indian women. In Indian Vedic (Hindu) religion, the Bindi highlights the "third" or "spiritual eye."

Chipko Movement: In India there is an ancient legend about a girl, Amrita Devi, who died trying to protect the trees that surrounded her village. The story recounts a time when the local maharajah's tree cutters arrived to cut down the villagers' trees for wood for his new fortress. Amrita, with others, jumped in front of the trees and hugged them, signifying protection.

Dal or *Dahl:* A thick, creamy East Indian stew made with lentils or other legumes, simmered with onions and various spices.

Dhanyawaad: Thank you

Dhobi wallahs: Indian residents who provide laundry service. They take the motel guests' laundry to wash, air-dry, press, fold and bundle before returning it to the motel. The secret behind this smooth operation is a symbol marked on each item of clothing; each dhobi wallah has his or her own code—invisible to the untrained eye but understood by all in the washing business—that ensures the safe passage of laundry.

Dosas: Food: A type of thin savory crepe from South India.

Dupatta: A long scarf traditionally worn by Indian women. It is often wrapped front to back over both shoulders.

Kal malenge: See you tomorrow.

Kurta: Tunic

Mandala: A ritualistic geometric design within a circle, symbolic of the universe, used in Hinduism and Buddhism as an aid to meditation.

Maph karna: Excuse me. I am sorry.

Namaste: Hello, good-bye, peace.

Nan or *naan:* A flat leavened bread of northwest India, made of white flour and baked in a tandoor oven.

Neem tree: Neem has two closely related species: *A. indica* A. Juss. and *M. azedarac*. The former is popularly known as Indian neem (margosa tree) or Indian lilac, and the other as the Persian lilac. Neem has been extensively used in ayurveda and homeopathic medicine. The Sanskrit name of the Neem tree is *Arishtha*, meaning "reliever of sickness." Each part of the Neem tree has some medicinal property.

Roti: An unleavened griddle-baked bread from India, usually made with whole wheat flour. The roti is finished over an open flame for 10 to 15 seconds, a technique that causes it to fill with steam and puff up like a balloon.

Thek hai: Fine, or good, or okay.

REFERENCES

Elie, Paul. 2003. *The Life You Save May Be Your Own: An American Pilgrimage.* New York: Farrar, Straus and Giroux.

Kidd, Sue Monk. 2002. *The Secret Life of Bees.* New York: Viking Penguin.

Macdonald, Sarah. 2002. *Holy Cow: An Indian Adventure.* Bantam Books: Sydney, Australia.

Melwani, Lavina. 2005. MRI tourists; Intrepid travelers to India are not headed for the Taj Mahal or the burning ghats of Benares, but for some of the best hospitals in India. *Little India,* April 30.

UNC Health Care looks at discounts. 2005. *The News and Observer* (Raleigh, NC), May 17, p. D1.